I0056726

IARC MONOGRAPHS

ON THE

EVALUATION OF THE CARCINOGENIC RISK

OF CHEMICALS TO MAN:

Some aziridines, *N-*, *S-* & *O-*mustards and selenium

Volume 9

This publication represents the views of an
IARC Working Group on the
Evaluation of the Carcinogenic Risk of Chemicals to Man
which met in Lyon,
8-14 April 1975

IARC WORKING GROUP ON THE EVALUATION OF THE CARCINOGENIC RISK OF CHEMICALS TO MAN: SOME AZIRIDINES, *N*-, *S*- AND *O*-MUSTARDS AND SELENIUM

Lyon, 8-14 April 1975

Members[1]

Mr H. Baxter, Laboratory of the Government Chemist, Cornwall House, Stamford Street, London SE1, UK

Professor E. Boyland, London School of Hygiene and Tropical Medicine, Keppel Street, London WC1E 7HT, UK (*Vice-Chairman*)

Dr I. Chernozemsky, Chief, Experimental Branch and Laboratory of Carcinogenesis, National Center of Oncology, Medical Academy, Sofia 56/Darvenitza, Bulgaria

Dr L. Kinlen, Department of the Regius Professor of Medicine, University of Oxford, Radcliffe Infirmary, Oxford OX2 6HE, UK

Dr P. Kleihues, Abteilung für Allgemeine Neurologie, Max-Planck Institut für Hirnforschung, Osterheimer Strasse 200, 5 Köln-Merheim, FRG

Dr H.V. Malling, Mutagenesis Branch, National Institute of Environmental Health Sciences, Research Triangle Park, North Carolina 27709, USA

Dr G. Mohn[2], Zentrallaboratorium für Mutagenitatsprüfung der Deutschen Forschungsgemeinschaft, Breisacher Strasse 33, 78 Freiburg, FRG

Dr P.J. O'Connor, Paterson Laboratories, Christie Hospital & Holt Radium Institute, Manchester M20 9BX, UK

Dr R. Saracci, Chief, Biostatistics & Clinical Epidemiology Section, CNR Laboratory for Clinical Physiology, University of Pisa, Via Savi 8, 56100 Pisa, Italy

Professor D. Schmähl, Direktor des Instituts für Toxikologie und Chemotherapie am Deutschen Krebsforschungszentrum, Im Neuenheimer Feld 280, 69 Heidelberg, FRG (*Chairman*)

---

[1]Unable to attend: Dr E. Arrhenius, Department of Environmental Toxicology, Stockholms Universitet, Wallenberglaboratoriet, Lilla Frescati, S 10405 Stockholm 50, Sweden

[2]On sabbatical leave during 1975 at the National Institute of Environmental Health Sciences, Environmental Mutagenesis Branch, Research Triangle Park, North Carolina 27709, USA

Dr R.J. Shamberger, The Clinic Center, Department of Biochemistry, Cleveland Clinic, 9500 Euclid Avenue, Cleveland, Ohio 44106, USA

Dr B. Teichmann, Akademie der Wissenschaften der DDR, Zentralinstitut für Krebsforschung, Lindenberger Weg 80, 1115 Berlin-Buch, GDR

Dr V.S. Turusov, Institute of Experimental and Clinical Oncology, Academy of Medical Sciences of the USSR, Karshirskoya Shosse 6, Moscow B-409, USSR

Professor F. Zajdela, Institut du Radium, Faculté des Sciences, Bâtiment 110, 91400 Orsay, France

Invited Guests

Dr R. Kroes, Head of the Department of Oncology, Laboratory for Pathology, Rijks Instituut voor de Volksgezondheid, Postbus 1, Bilthoven, The Netherlands

Dr R.H. Reinfried, Stanford Research Institute, Pelikanstrasse 37, 8001 Zurich, Switzerland

Mr D.E. Schendel, Industrial Economist, Chemical Information Services, Stanford Research Institute, Menlo Park, California 94025, USA (*Rapporteur sections 2.1 and 2.2*)

Representative from the National Cancer Institute

Dr Marcia Litwack, Carcinogenesis DCCP, National Cancer Institute, Bethesda, Maryland 20014, USA

Secretariat

Dr C. Agthe, Unit of Chemical Carcinogenesis (*Secretary*)

Dr H. Bartsch, Unit of Chemical Carcinogenesis (*Rapporteur section 3.2*)

Dr L. Griciute, Chief, Unit of Environmental Carcinogens

Dr G. Margison, Unit of Chemical Carcinogenesis

Dr B. Marschall, Occupational Health, WHO

Dr R. Montesano, Unit of Chemical Carcinogenesis (*Rapporteur section 3.1*)

Mrs C. Partensky, Unit of Chemical Carcinogenesis (*Technical editor*)

Dr V. Ponomarkov, Unit of Chemical Carcinogenesis

Dr L. Tomatis, Chief, Unit of Chemical Carcinogenesis (*Head of the Programme*)

Dr A. Tuyns, Unit of Epidemiology and Biostatistics (*Rapporteur section 3.3*)

Mr E.A. Walker, Unit of Environmental Carcinogens (*Rapporteur section 2.3*)

Mrs E. Ward, Montignac, France (*Editor*)

Mr J.D. Wilbourn, Unit of Chemical Carcinogenesis (*Co-secretary*)

Note to the reader

Every effort is made to present the monographs as accurately as possible without unduly delaying their publication. Nevertheless, mistakes have occurred and are still likely to occur. In the interest of all users of these monographs, readers are requested to communicate any errors observed to the Unit of Chemical Carcinogenesis of the International Agency for Research on Cancer, Lyon, France, in order that these can be included in corrigenda which will appear in subsequent volumes.

As stated in the preamble, great efforts are made to cover the whole literature, but some studies may have been inadvertently overlooked. Since the monographs are not intended to be a review of the literature and contain only data considered relevant by the Working Group, it is not possible for the reader to determine whether a certain study was considered or not. However, research workers who are aware of important published data which may change the evaluation are requested to make them available to the above-mentioned address, in order that they can be considered for a possible re-evaluation by a future Working Group.

CONTENTS

BACKGROUND AND PURPOSE OF THE IARC PROGRAMME ON THE EVALUATION
OF THE CARCINOGENIC RISK OF CHEMICALS TO MAN 11

SCOPE OF THE MONOGRAPHS 11

MECHANISM FOR PRODUCING THE MONOGRAPHS 12

    Priority for the preparation of monographs 12

    Data on which the evaluation is based 12

    The Working Group 13

GENERAL PRINCIPLES FOR THE EVALUATION 13

    Terminology 13

    Response to carcinogens 14

    Purity of the compounds tested 14

    Qualitative aspects 14

    Quantitative aspects 15

    Animal data in relation to the evaluation of risk to man 15

    Evidence of human carcinogenicity 15

EXPLANATORY NOTES ON THE MONOGRAPHS 16

GENERAL REMARKS ON THE SUBSTANCES CONSIDERED 25

THE MONOGRAPHS

    Aziridines:

        Apholate 31

        Aziridine 37

        2-(1-Aziridinyl)ethanol 47

        Aziridyl benzoquinone 51

        Bis(1-aziridinyl)morpholinophosphine sulphide 55

        2-Methylaziridine 61

        Tris(aziridinyl)-*para*-benzoquinone 67

        Tris(1-aziridinyl)phosphine oxide 75

        Tris(1-aziridinyl)phosphine sulphide 85

        2,4,6-Tris(1-aziridinyl)-*s*-triazine 95

        Tris(2-methyl-1-aziridinyl)phosphine oxide 107

Mustards:

Bis(2-chloroethyl)ether 117

Chlorambucil 125

Cyclophosphamide 135

Mannomustine (dihydrochloride) 157

Melphalan, medphalan and merphalan 167

Mustard gas 181

Nitrogen mustard (hydrochloride) 193

Nitrogen mustard *N*-oxide (hydrochloride)................... 209

Oestradiol mustard 217

Phenoxybenzamine (hydrochloride) 223

Trichlorotriethylamine hydrochloride 229

Uracil mustard 235

Selenium and selenium compounds 245

CUMULATIVE INDEX TO MONOGRAPHS 261

BACKGROUND AND PURPOSE OF THE IARC PROGRAMME ON THE
EVALUATION OF THE CARCINOGENIC RISK OF CHEMICALS TO MAN

The International Agency for Research on Cancer (IARC) initiated in 1971 a programme on the evaluation of the carcinogenic risk of chemicals to man. This programme was supported by a Resolution of the Governing Council at its Ninth Session concerning the role of IARC in providing government authorities with expert, independent scientific opinion on environmental carcinogenesis. As one means to this end, the Governing Council recommended that IARC should continue to prepare monographs on the carcinogenic risk of individual chemicals to man.

In view of the importance of this programme and in order to expedite the production of monographs, the National Cancer Institute of the United States has provided IARC with additional funds for this purpose.

The objective of this programme is to elaborate and publish in the form of monographs a critical review of carcinogenicity and related data in the light of the present state of knowledge, with the final aim of evaluating the data in terms of possible human risk, and at the same time to indicate where additional research efforts are needed.

SCOPE OF THE MONOGRAPHS

The monographs summarize the evidence for the carcinogenicity of individual chemicals and other relevant information. The data are compiled, reviewed and evaluated by a Working Group of experts. No recommendations are given concerning preventive measures or legislation, since these matters depend on risk-benefit evaluation, which seems best made by individual governments and/or international agencies such as WHO and ILO.

Since 1973, when the programme was started, eight volumes have been published[1,2,3,4,5,6,7,8].

As new data on chemicals for which monographs have already been written and new principles for evaluation become available, re-evaluations will be made at future meetings, and revised monographs will be published as necessary. The monographs are being distributed to international and governmental agencies and will be available to industries and scientists dealing with these chemicals. They also form the basis of advice from IARC on carcinogenesis from these substances.

MECHANISM FOR PRODUCING THE MONOGRAPHS

As a first step, a list of chemicals for possible consideration by the Working Group is established. IARC then collects pertinent references regarding physico-chemical characteristics, production and use*, occurrence and analysis, and biological data** on these compounds. The material is summarized by an expert consultant or an IARC staff member, who prepares the first draft, which in some cases is sent to another expert for comments. The drafts are circulated to all members of the Working Group about one month before the meeting. During the meeting further additions to and deletions from the data are agreed upon, and a final version of comments and evaluation on each compound is adopted.

Priority for the Preparation of Monographs

Priority is given mainly to chemicals belonging to groups for which at least some suggestion of carcinogenicity exists from observations in animals and/or man and for which there is evidence of human exposure. However, neither human exposure nor potential carcinogenicity can be judged until all the relevant data have been collected and examined in detail, and the inclusion of a particular compound in a monograph does not necessarily mean that the substance is considered to be carcinogenic. Equally, the fact that a substance has not yet been considered does not imply that it is without carcinogenic hazard.

Data on which the Evaluation is Based

With regard to the biological data, only published articles and papers already accepted for publication are reviewed. Every effort is made to

----

*Data provided by Chemical Information Services, Stanford Research Institute, Menlo Park, California, USA

**In the collection of original data reference was made to the publications "Survey of compounds which have been tested for carcinogenic activity"[9,10,11,12,13,14].

cover the whole literature, but some studies may have been inadvertently overlooked. The monographs are not intended to be a full review of the literature, and they contain only data considered relevant by the Group. Research workers who are aware of important data (published or accepted for publication) which may influence the evaluation are invited to make them available to the Unit of Chemical Carcinogenesis of the International Agency for Research on Cancer, Lyon, France.

The Working Group

The tasks of the Working Group are five-fold: (1) to verify that as far as feasible all data have been collected; (2) to select the data relevant for the evaluation; (3) to determine whether the data, as summarized, will enable the reader to follow the reasoning of the committee; (4) to judge the significance of the experimental results; and (5) to make an evaluation.

The members of the Working Group who participated in the consideration of particular substances are listed at the beginning of each publication. The members of the Working Group serve in their individual capacities as scientists, and not as representatives of their governments or of any organization with which they are affiliated.

GENERAL PRINCIPLES FOR THE EVALUATION

The general principles for the evaluation which are listed below were elaborated by previous Working Groups and were also applied to the substances listed in this volume.

Terminology

The term "chemical carcinogenesis" in its widely accepted sense is used to indicate the induction or enhancement of neoplasia by chemicals. It is recognized that, in the strict etymological sense, this term means the induction of cancer; however, common usage has led to its employment to denote the induction of various types of neoplasms. The terms "tumourigen", "oncogen" and "blastomogen" have all been used synonymously with "carcinogen", although occasionally "tumourigen" has been used specifically to denote the induction of benign tumours.

Response to Carcinogens

For present purposes, in general, no distinction is made between the induction of tumours and the enhancement of tumour incidence, although it is noted that there may be fundamental differences in mechanisms that will eventually be elucidated.

The response in experimental animals to a carcinogen may take several forms:

(1) a significant increase in the incidence of one or more of the same types of neoplasms as found in control animals;

(2) the occurrence of types of neoplasms not observed in control animals;

(3) a decreased latent period as compared with control animals.

Purity of the Compounds Tested

In any evaluation of biological data with respect to a possible carcinogenic risk, particular attention must be paid to the purity of the chemicals tested and to their stability under conditions of storage or administration. Information on purity and stability is given, when available, in the monographs.

Qualitative Aspects

The qualitative nature of neoplasia has been much discussed. In many instances, both benign and malignant tumours are induced by chemical carcinogens. There are so far few recorded instances in which only benign tumours are induced by chemicals that have been studied extensively. Their occurrence in experimental systems has been taken to indicate the possibility of an increased risk of malignant tumours also.

In experimental carcinogenesis, the type of cancer seen can be the same as that recorded in human studies (e.g., bladder cancer in man, monkeys, dogs and hamsters after administration of 2-naphthylamine). In other instances, however, a chemical can induce other types of neoplasms or neoplasms at different sites in various species (e.g., benzidine induces hepatic carcinoma in the rat, but bladder carcinoma in man).

14

Quantitative Aspects

Dose-response studies are important in the evaluation of human and animal carcinogenesis. The confidence with which a carcinogenic effect can be established is strengthened by the observation of an increasing incidence of neoplasms with increasing exposure. Such studies are the only ones on which a minimal effective dose can be established. The determination of such a dose allows a comparison with reliable data on human exposure.

Comparison of potency between compounds can only be made if and when substances have been tested simultaneously.

Animal Data in Relation to the Evaluation of Risk to Man

At the present time no attempt can be made to interpret the animal data directly in terms of human risk since no objective criteria are available to do so. The critical assessment of the validity of the animal data given in these monographs is intended to assist national and/or international authorities to make decisions concerning preventive measures or legislation. In this connection attention is drawn to WHO recommendations in relation to food additives[15], drugs[16] and occupational carcinogens[17].

Evidence of Human Carcinogenicity

Evaluation of the carcinogenic risk to man of suspected environmental agents rests on purely observational studies. Such studies require sufficient variation in the levels of human exposure to allow a meaningful relationship between cancer incidence and exposure to a given chemical to be established. Difficulties in isolating the effects of individual agents arise, however, since populations are exposed to multiple carcinogens.

The initial suggestion of a relationship between an agent and disease often comes from case reports of patients who have had similar exposures. Variations and time trends in regional or national cancer incidence, or their correlation with regional or national 'exposure' levels, may also provide valuable insights. Such observations by themselves, however, cannot in most circumstances be regarded as conclusive evidence of carcinogenicity. The most satisfactory epidemiological method is to compare the cancer risk (adjusted for age, sex and other confounding variables) among groups or cohorts, or among individuals exposed to various levels of the agent in question, and among control groups not so exposed. Ideally this is accomplished directly, by following such groups forward in time (prospectively) to determine time relationships, dose-response relationships and other aspects of cancer induction. Large cohorts and long observation periods are required to provide sufficient cases for a statistically valid comparison.

An alternative to prospective investigation is to assemble cohorts from past records and to evaluate their subsequent morbidity or mortality by means of medical histories and death certificates. Such occupational carcinogens as nickel, β-naphthylamine, asbestos and benzidine have been confirmed by this method. Another method is to compare the past exposures of a defined group of cancer cases with those of control samples from the hospital or general population. This does not provide an absolute measure of carcinogenic risk but can indicate the relative risks associated with different levels of exposure. The indirect means (e.g., interviews or tissue residues) used to measure exposures which may have commenced many years before can constitute a major source of error. Nevertheless such "case-control" studies can often isolate one factor from several suspected agents. The carcinogenic effect of this substance could then be confirmed by cohort studies.

EXPLANATORY NOTES ON THE MONOGRAPHS

In sections 1, 2 and 3 of each monograph, except for minor remarks, the data are recorded as given by the author, whereas the comments by the Working Group are given in section 4, headed "Comments on Data Reported and Evaluation".

Chemical and Physical Data (section 1)

The Chemical Abstracts Registry Serial Number and the latest Chemical Abstracts Name (if this is not used in the title) are recorded in this section, together with other synonyms and trade names.

Chemical and physical properties include data that might be relevant to carcinogenicity (for example, lipid solubility) and those that concern identification. Where applicable, data on solubility, volatility and stability are indicated. All chemical data in this section refer to the pure substance.

Production, Use, Occurrence and Analysis (section 2)

The ultimate purpose of this section is to give an idea of the extent of possible human exposure, and therefore data on production, use and occurrence are given when available. With regard to these data, IARC has collaborated with the Stanford Research Institute, USA, with the support of the National Cancer Institute of the USA, in order to obtain production figures of chemicals and their patterns of use.

Since the United States, Western Europe and Japan are reasonably representative industrialized areas, and since Stanford Research Institute has regional offices in these areas, such data are commonly acquired from these countries. It should not be inferred that these nations are the sole sources or even the major sources of any individual chemical.

Production data are obtained from both governmental and trade publications in the three geographic areas. Information on use and occurrence is obtained by a comprehensive review of published data, complemented by direct contact with manufacturers of the chemicals in question.

Since cancer is a delayed toxic effect, past use and production data are also of importance. With respect to past and present use and production, regulatory actions in some countries are mentioned as examples only. Statements concerning regulations may not reflect the most recent situation, since such legislation is in a constant state of change; nor should it be taken to imply that other countries do not have similar regulations. In the cases of drugs, mention of the therapeutic uses of such chemicals does not necessarily represent presently accepted therapeutic indications, nor does it imply judgement as to their clinical efficacy.

It is hoped that in future revisions of these monographs, more information on production and use can be made available to IARC from other countries.

17

Biological Data Relevant to the Evaluation of Carcinogenic
Risk to Man (section 3)

As pointed out earlier in this introduction, the monographs are not
intended to consider all reported studies. Although every effort was made
to review the whole literature, some studies were purposely omitted (a)
because of their inadequacy, as judged from previously described criteria
[18,19,20,21] (e.g., too short a duration, too few animals, poor survival or
too small a dose); (b) because they only confirmed findings which have
already been fully described; or (c) because they were judged irrelevant
for the purpose of the evaluation. However, in certain cases, reference is
made to studies which did not meet established criteria of adequacy, particularly when this information was considered a useful supplement to other
reports or when it may have been the only data available. This does not,
however, imply acceptance of the adequacy of experimental designs in these
cases.

In general, the data recorded in this section are summarized as given
by the author; however, certain shortcomings of reporting or of experimental design are also mentioned, and minor comments by the Working Group
are given in square brackets.

The essential comments by the Working Group are made in section 4,
"Comments on Data Reported and Evaluation".

Carcinogenicity and related studies in animals: Mention is usually
made of all routes of administration by which the compound has been tested
and of all species in which relevant tests have been carried out. In most
cases the animal strains are given; general characteristics of mouse strains
have been reported in a recent review[22]. Quantitative data are given in so
far as they will enable the reader to realize the order of magnitude of the
effective doses. In general, the doses are indicated as they appear in the
original paper; sometimes conversions have been made for better comparison.

Other relevant biological data: The reporting of metabolic data is
restricted to studies showing the metabolic fate of the chemical in animals
and man. Comparison of animal and human data is made when possible. Other
metabolic information (e.g., absorption, storage and excretion) is given

when the Working Group considered that it would enable the reader to have a better understanding of the fate of the compound in the body. When the carcinogenicity of known metabolites has been tested, this also is reported.

Some LD_{50}'s are given, and other data on toxicity are included occasionally, if considered relevant.

Mutagenicity data are also included and the reasons for including such data and the principles adopted by the Working Group for selection of the data are outlined below.

Most of the chemical carcinogens which have so far been studied have been shown to require metabolic activation in order to produce their biological effects. This metabolic activation is in many cases associated with binding to nucleophilic sites in nucleic acids and proteins. The growing experimental evidence linking the carcinogenic activity of numerous chemicals to their capacity to be converted into electrophilic derivatives that may also exert a mutagenic effect has led to the suggestion that a relationship between chemical carcinogenesis and mutagenesis may exist. Such a correlation has so far been limited to those changes of the genotype which appear as a consequence of structural or functional alterations of nucleic acids.

Although not all chemical mutagens have been shown to be carcinogenic, most chemical carcinogens, several of which cause cancer in man, have now been found to be mutagens when tested in one of the mutagenicity test procedures that combine microbial, mammalian or other animal-cell systems as genetic targets with an *in vitro* or *in vivo* metabolic activation system. The results of appropriate mutagenicity tests, which are relatively rapid and inexpensive, may help to prescreen chemicals and may also aid in the selection of the most relevant animal species in which to carry out long-term carcinogenicity tests on these chemicals. The use of human tissues in such *in vitro* testing procedures allows correlations between experimental animals and humans to be made. For all these reasons, the Working Group decided to consider data on mutagenicity as relevant biological information to be included in the monographs.

There are many genetic indicators and metabolic activation systems available for detecting mutagenic activity; they all, however, have individual advantages and limitations. Ideally, an appropriate mutagenicity test system would include the full metabolic competency of the intact human. Since the development or application of such a system appears to be impossible, the conclusion has been reached that a battery of test systems is needed in order to detect the mutagenic potential of chemicals.

In many cases, reactive metabolites with a limited life-span may fail to reach or to react with the genetic indicator, either because they are further metabolized to inactive compounds or because they react with other cellular constituents. For this reason mutagenicity assays in intact animals may give false-negative results, and appropriate *in vitro* techniques involving organ perfusion, tissue slices, cultured cell lines or tissue fractions should be included in screening programmes. Useful information may also be provided by investigation of other biological functions relevant to carcinogenesis in humans, such as enzymes involved in the metabolic conversion of chemicals, DNA repair in human cells and immunological surveillance mechanisms.

Metabolism in mammals is affected by exogenous and endogenous factors, such as chemicals causing enzyme induction and inhibition, diet and gastrointestinal flora. Other factors should also be considered in the experimental design, e.g., age, sex and strain of animals, diurnal and seasonal rhythms, differences between the foetal and adult states and mode of administration, cellular uptake, distribution and excretion of the chemical. Differences in the metabolism of foreign compounds by *in vitro* preparations and by intact animals should also be taken into account. In view of all these factors, an incomplete picture of the mutagenic effects of chemical carcinogens *in vivo* may be obtained by *in vitro* techniques.

It is difficult in the present state of knowledge to select specific mutagenicity tests as being the most appropriate for the pre-screening of substances for possible carcinogenic activity. In deciding which mutagenicity test procedures should be used, preference should be given to systems that are genetically and metabolically reasonably well defined and/or which provide data shown to be valid for the prediction of the

20

carcinogenicity of chemicals. Consideration of the results (positive or negative) of mutagenicity tests using chemicals and their identified metabolites should be of great value in assessing the reliability of the correlation between carcinogenic and mutagenic activities of chemicals.

For more detailed information see references 23-28.

Observations in man: Epidemiological studies are summarized. Clinical and other observations in man have been reviewed, when relevant.

Comments on Data Reported and Evaluation (section 4)

This section gives the critical view of the Working Group on the data reported. It should be read in conjunction with the "General Remarks on the Substances Considered".

Animal data: The animal species mentioned are those in which the carcinogenicity of the substances was clearly demonstrated, irrespective of the route of administration. In the case of inadequate studies, when mentioned, comments to that effect are included. The route of administration used in experimental animals that is similar to the possible human exposure (ingestion, inhalation and skin exposure) is given particular mention. In most cases tumour sites are also indicated. Experiments involving a possible action of the vehicle or a physical effect of the agent, such as in subcutaneous injection or bladder implantation studies, are also mentioned; however, the results of such tests require careful consideration, particularly if they are the only ones raising a suspicion of carcinogenicity. If the substance has produced tumours on pre-natal exposure or in single-dose experiments, this is also indicated. This sub-section should be read in the light of comments made in the section "Animal Data in Relation to the Evaluation of Risk to Man" of this introduction.

Human data: In some cases, a brief statement is made on the possible exposure of man. The significance of epidemiological studies and case reports is discussed, and the data are interpreted in terms of possible human risk.

References

1. IARC (1972) IARC Monographs on the Evaluation of Carcinogenic Risk of Chemicals to Man, 1, Lyon

2. IARC (1973) IARC Monographs on the Evaluation of Carcinogenic Risk of Chemicals to Man, 2, Some Inorganic and Organometallic Compounds, Lyon

3. IARC (1973) IARC Monographs on the Evaluation of Carcinogenic Risk of Chemicals to Man, 3, Certain Polycyclic Aromatic Hydrocarbons and Heterocyclic Compounds, Lyon

4. IARC (1974) IARC Monographs on the Evaluation of Carcinogenic Risk of Chemicals to Man, 4, Some Aromatic Amines, Hydrazine and Related Substances, N-Nitroso Compounds and Miscellaneous Alkylating Agents, Lyon

5. IARC (1974) IARC Monographs on the Evaluation of Carcinogenic Risk of Chemicals to Man, 5, Some Organochlorine Pesticides, Lyon

6. IARC (1974) IARC Monographs on the Evaluation of Carcinogenic Risk of Chemicals to Man, 6, Sex Hormones, Lyon

7. IARC (1974) IARC Monographs on the Evaluation of Carcinogenic Risk of Chemicals to Man, 7, Some Anti-thyroid and Related Substances, Nitrofurans and Industrial Chemicals, Lyon

8. IARC (1975) IARC Monographs on the Evaluation of Carcinogenic Risk of Chemicals to Man, 8, Some Aromatic Azo Compounds, Lyon

9. Hartwell, J.L. (1951) Survey of compounds which have been tested for carcinogenic activity, Washington DC, US Government Printing Office (Public Health Service Publication No. 149)

10. Shubik, P. & Hartwell, J.L. (1957) Survey of compounds which have been tested for carcinogenic activity, Washington DC, US Government Printing Office (Public Health Service Publication No. 149: Supplement 1)

11. Shubik, P. & Hartwell, J.L. (1969) Survey of compounds which have been tested for carcinogenic activity, Washington DC, US Government Printing Office (Public Health Service Publication No. 149: Supplement 2)

12. Carcinogenesis Program National Cancer Institute (1971) Survey of compounds which have been tested for carcinogenic activity, Washington DC, US Government Printing Office (Public Health Service Publication No. 149: 1968-1969)

13. Carcinogenesis Program National Cancer Institute (1973) _Survey of compounds which have been tested for carcinogenic activity_, Washington DC, US Government Printing Office (Public Health Service Publication No. 149: 1961-1967)

14. Carcinogenesis Program National Cancer Institute (1974) _Survey of compounds which have been tested for carcinogenic activity_, Washington DC, US Government Printing Office (Public Health Service Publication No. 149: 1970-1971)

15. WHO (1961) Fifth Report of the Joint FAO/WHO Expert Committee on Food Additives. Evaluation of carcinogenic hazard of food additives. _Wld Hlth Org. techn. Rep. Ser._, No. 220, pp. 5, 18, 19

16. WHO (1969) Report of a WHO Scientific Group. Principles for the testing and evaluation of drugs for carcinogenicity. _Wld Hlth Org. techn. Rep. Ser._, No. 426, pp. 19, 21, 22

17. WHO (1964) Report of a WHO Expert Committee. Prevention of cancer. _Wld Hlth Org. techn. Rep. Ser._, No. 276, pp. 29, 30

18. WHO (1958) Second Report of the Joint FAO/WHO Expert Committee on Food Additives. Procedures for the testing of intentional food additives to establish their safety for use. _Wld Hlth Org. techn. Rep. Ser._, No. 144

19. WHO (1961) Fifth Report of the Joint FAO/WHO Expert Committee on Food Additives. Evaluation of carcinogenic hazard of food additives. _Wld Hlth Org. techn. Rep. Ser._, No. 220

20. WHO (1967) Scientific Group. Procedures for investigating intentional and unintentional food additives. _Wld Hlth Org. techn. Rep. Ser._, No. 348

21. UICC (1969) Carcinogenicity testing. _UICC techn. Rep. Ser._, 2

22. Committee on Standardized Genetic Nomenclature for Mice (1972) Standardized nomenclature for inbred strains of mice. Fifth listing. _Cancer Res._, 32, 1609-1646

23. Bartsch, H. & Grover, P.L. (1974) _Chemical carcinogenesis and mutagenesis_. In: Symington, T. & Carter, R.L., eds, _Scientific Foundations of Oncology_, Vol. IX, _Chemical Carcinogenesis_, London, Heinemann Medical Books Ltd (in press)

24. Holländer, A., ed. (1971) _Chemical Mutagens: Principles and Methods for Their Detection_, Vols 1-3, New York, Plenum Press

25. Montesano, R. & Tomatis, L., eds (1974) Chemical Carcinogenesis Essays, _IARC Scientific Publications_, No. 10, Lyon, IARC

26. Ramel, C., ed. (1973) Evaluation of genetic risks of environmental
        chemicals, Report of a symposium held at Skokloster, Sweden,
        1972, Ambio Special Report No. 3, Royal Swedish Academy of
        Sciences/Universitetsforlaget

27. Stoltz, D.R., Poirier, L.A., Irving, C.C., Stich, H.F., Weisburger,
        J.H. & Grice, H.C. (1974) Evaluation of short-term tests for
        carcinogenicity. Toxicol. appl. Pharmacol., 29, 157-180

28. WHO (1974) Report of a WHO Scientific Group. Assessment of the
        carcinogenicity and mutagenicity of chemicals. Wld Hlth Org.
        techn. Rep. Ser., No. 546

GENERAL REMARKS ON THE SUBSTANCES CONSIDERED

The substances considered in this volume, with the exception of selenium compounds, are direct or indirect alkylating agents having a variety of biological and therapeutic effects, including cytostatic and immunosuppressive activities. Some are drugs and have been used and are used in the treatment of neoplastic and non-neoplastic disorders in man.

The chemistry, metabolism and biological effects of alkylating agents have been reported in several reviews (Jones, 1973; Lawley, 1974; Loveless, 1966; Ross, 1962; Van Duuren, 1969; Wheeler, 1962).

A cytotoxic effect on dividing cells is the characteristic pharmacological action of alkylating agents and the basis of their use as anti-cancer drugs. This is associated with an inactivation of the DNA template by the formation of single strand breaks and interstrand crosslinks, in the case of bifunctional alkylating agents, which results in an inhibition of DNA synthesis. Toxic effects on resting cells also occur, but the dose required is higher. Alkylating compounds cause preferential damage to organs which have a high rate of cell turnover.

Lethal doses typically attack dividing cells. When given to animals, alkylating agents also exert cytotoxic effects on the embryo. The resultant teratogenic effects depend largely on the stage of foetal development and the extent to which the compound or its active metabolites pass the placental barrier.

In addition to inactivation of the DNA template, some alkylating agents produce lesions which affect base-pairing during DNA replication and cause permanent genetic alterations. All alkylating agents must be regarded as potential carcinogens and mutagens.

The development of tumours following exposure to some of these substances could be due to a direct chemical action or to impairment of the immune system or to both (Doll & Kinlen, 1970; Gilbert, 1972; Good, 1973; Kripke & Borsos, 1974; Kroes *et al.*, 1975; Krüger, 1974; Leibowitz & Schwartz, 1971; Penn, 1974).

Since many of these substances have been shown to cause cancer in animals, the possibility must be considered that they have a similar effect in man. However, with the exception of studies of men exposed to mustard gas and a current prospective study of patients treated with certain of these drugs for non-malignant disorders (Cameron, 1975; Doll & Kinlen, 1970), available human data on cancer in relation to the aziridines or mustards are restricted to case reports. These refer mainly to the occurrence of second primary neoplasms (in some instances after only a short interval) following their use, often in combination, in the treatment of malignant diseases, although tumours have also been reported after their use in non-malignant diseases. The problem is to decide if the incidence is increased. Although the occurrence of multiple primary neoplasms was known before the introduction of such drugs, reports concerning their association with chemotherapy are to be expected, particularly in view of the increased survival of cancer patients achieved by these means. Evaluation of second primary tumours is a difficult epidemiological problem, whatever the treatment. There is, however, a dearth of population studies that have compared the incidence of second primary tumours in patients receiving chemotherapy with that in patients who did not receive such treatment, taking appropriate account of the person-years of experience after diagnosis of the first cancer.

From a practical standpoint one should not forget that the risk-benefit balance when prescribing a drug which carries a carcinogenic risk is likely to be remarkably different in the treatment of fatal conditions like cancer, especially when no effective alternative treatment is available, from that in non-cancerous conditions, especially if alternative forms of treatment are available.

Selenium was considered by this Working Group in view of the forthcoming WHO Environmental Health Criteria document on this substance.

References

Cameron, J.S. (1975) Problems with immunosuppressive agents in renal disease. J. clin. Path., 28, suppl. 9 (in press)

Doll, R. & Kinlen, L. (1970) Immunosurveillance and cancer: epidemiological evidence. Brit. med. J., iv, 420-422

Gilbert, J.R., ed. (1972) Conference on immunology of carcinogenesis. Nat. Cancer Inst. Monogr., 35, 1-477

Good, R.A. (1973) Immunodeficiency and malignancy. In: Doll, R. & Vodopija, I., eds, Host Environment Interactions in the Etiology of Cancer in Man, Lyon, IARC, pp. 265-274

Jones, A.R. (1973) The metabolism of biological alkylating agents. In: Di Carlo, F.J., ed., Drug Metabolism Reviews, Vol. 2, New York, Dekker, pp. 71-100

Kripke, M.L. & Borsos, T. (1974) Immunosuppression and carcinogenesis. A review. Israel J. med. Sci., 10, 888

Kroes, R., Weiss, J.W. & Weisburger, J.H. (1975) Immunosuppression and chemical carcinogenesis. Recent Results Cancer Res. (in press)

Krüger, G.R.F. (1974) Lymphoreticular neoplasia in immunosuppression: facts and fancies. Beitr. path. Anat., 151, 221-223

Lawley, P.D. (1974) Some chemical aspects of dose-response relationships in alkylation mutagenesis. Mutation Res., 23, 283-295

Leibowitz, S. & Schwartz, R.S. (1971) Malignancy as a complication of immunosuppressive therapy. Advanc. int. Med., 17, 95-123

Loveless, A. (1966) Genetic and Allied Effects of Alkylating Agents, London, Butterworths

Penn, I. (1974) Chemical immunosuppression and human cancer. Cancer, 34, 1474-1480

Ross, W.C.J. (1962) Biological Alkylating Agents: Fundamental Chemistry and the Design of Compounds for Selective Toxicity, London, Butterworths

Van Duuren, B.L. (1969) Biological effects of alkylating agents. Ann. N.Y. Acad. Sci., 163, 589-1029

Wheeler, G.P. (1962) Studies related to the mechanism of action of cytotoxic alkylating agents: A review. Cancer Res., 22, 651-687

AZIRIDINES

APHOLATE

1. Chemical and Physical Data

1.1 Synonyms and trade names

Chem. Abstr. Reg. Serial No.:   52-46-0

Chem. Abstr. Name: 2,2,4,4,6,6-Hexakis(1-aziridinyl)-2,2,4,4,6,6-
hexahydro-1,3,5,2,4,6-triazatriphosphorine

APN;   aziridine, 1,3,5,2,4-6-triazatriphosphorine derivative;
1-aziridinylphosphonitrile trimer;   ENT 26,316;   hexa(1-aziridinyl)-
triphosphotriazine;   2,2,4,4,6,6-hexakis(1-aziridinyl)cyclotri-
phosphaza-1,3,5-triene;   2,2,4,4,5,5-hexakis(1-aziridinyl)-2,2,4,4,5,5-
hexahydro-1,3,5,2,4,6-triazatriphosphorine;   hexakis(aziridinyl)-
phosphotriazine

1.2 Chemical formula and molecular weight

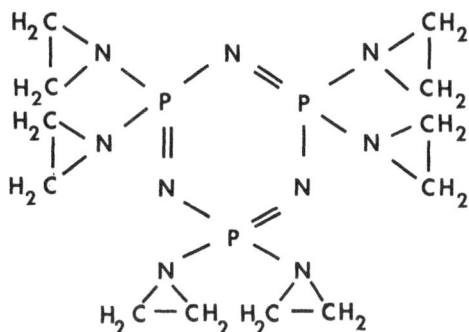

$C_{12}H_{24}N_9P_3$

Mol. wt: 387.3

1.3 Chemical and physical properties of the pure substance

(a) Description: Crystals (from heptane)

(b) Melting-point: 147.5°C (crystallized from heptane) (Stecher,
1968);   154-154.5°C (crystallized from ethylacetate) (Bowman &
Beroza, 1966)

(c) Spectroscopy data: Infra-red (Rätz *et al.*, 1964);   NMR
(Ottmann *et al.*, 1964)

1.4 Technical products and impurities

No data were available to the Working Group.

2. Production, Use, Occurrence and Analysis

For important background information on this section, see preamble, p. 17.

2.1 Production and use

Apholate can be prepared by the addition of aziridine to 2,2,4,4,6,6-hexachloro-2,2,4,4,5,5-hexahydrotriazatriphosphorine (Rätz & Grundmann, 1958); however, it has been produced for research purposes only.

Apholate has been tested as an antineoplastic agent (Chernov *et al.*, 1959), but it does not appear to have been used for this purpose in human medicine. It has been shown to be an effective chemosterilant for various insects (LaBrecque, 1961; Smith *et al.*, 1964), but problems associated with its application to insects, its toxicity and possible environmental effects have prevented its use in this way on a commercial basis.

2.2 Occurrence

Apholate is not known to occur in nature.

2.3 Analysis

Analytical methods for the estimation of apholate include titrimetry, colorimetry and thin-layer chromatography (Beroza & Borkovec, 1964). Following its extraction from biological material, 0.1 ng apholate can be detected by gas chromatography (Bowman & Beroza, 1966).

3. Biological Data Relevant to the Evaluation of Carcinogenic Risk to Man

3.1 Carcinogenicity and related studies in animals

Oral administration

Rat: Sixty weanling male and female Fischer rats received apholate in steroid-suspending vehicle*, by gavage, on 5 days per week in daily doses per animal of 0.003-0.1 mg (12 males and 12 females), 0.3 mg (15 males and 15 females) or 1 mg (maximum tolerated dose, given to 3 males and 3 females) for up to 1 year. Average survival times ranged from 340 days in males given the highest dose to 565 days in females given the lowest dose. The tumour incidence was reported to be similar to that in controls; no tumours were reported to have occurred in animals given the highest dose level (Hadidian *et al.*, 1968). [The small number of animals used should be noted.]

3.2 Other relevant biological data

The oral LD_{50}'s of apholate for male and female Sherman rats were found to be 98 and 113 mg/kg bw. The LD_{50} by skin application was 400-800 mg/kg bw for rats of both sexes (Gaines, 1969; Gaines & Kimbrough, 1964).

Treatment of *Neurospora conidia* with apholate induced an increase in the frequency of recessive lethal mutations (Kaney & Atwood, 1964). After i.p. injection of 1.5 mg/kg bw apholate into mice, a peak of chromosome and chromatid aberrations was found in the bone marrow 24 hours later (Manna & Das, 1973). Treatment of cultured human lymphocytes for 8 hours with apholate produced 89% abnormal cells with 2.6 gaps or breaks per cell (Chang & Klassen, 1968).

3.3 Observations in man

No data were available to the Working Group.

4. Comments on Data Reported and Evaluation

4.1 Animal data

In the only available study, apholate was inadequately tested by the oral route in rats; no evaluation on the carcinogenicity of this chemical can be made.

---

*NaCl, Na carboxymethylcellulose, Polysorbate 80, benzyl alcohol and water

4.2 Human data

No case reports or epidemiological studies were available to the Working Group.

5. References

Beroza, M. & Borkovec, A.B. (1964) Stability of tepa [tris-(1-aziridinyl)-phosphine oxide] and other aziridine chemosterilants. J. med. Chem., 7, 44-49

Bowman, M.C. & Beroza, M. (1966) Gas chromatographic determination of trace amounts of the insect chemosterilants tepa, metepa, methiotepa, hempa and apholate and the analysis of tepa in insect tissue. J. Ass. off. analyt. Chem., 49, 1046-1052

Chang, T.H. & Klassen, W. (1968) Comparative effects of tretamine, tepa, apholate and their structural analogs on human chromosomes *in vitro*. Chromosoma (Berl.), 24, 314-323

Chernov, V.A., Lytkina, V.B., Sergievskaya, S.I., Kropacheva, A.A., Parshina, V.A. & Sventsitskaya, L.E. (1959) Antitumor activity of some phosphonitrile trimer and tetramer derivatives. Farmakol. i Toksikol., 22, 365-367

Gaines, T.B. (1969) Acute toxicity of pesticides. Toxicol. appl. Pharmacol., 14, 515-534

Gaines, T.B. & Kimbrough, R.D. (1964) Toxicity of metepa to rats with notes on two other chemosterilants. Bull. Wld Hlth Org., 31, 737-745

Hadidian, Z., Fredrickson, T.N., Weisburger, E.K., Weisburger, J.H., Glass, R.M. & Mantel, N. (1968) Tests for chemical carcinogens. Report on the activity of derivatives of aromatic amines, nitrosamines, quinolines, nitroalkanes, amides, epoxides, aziridines and purine antimetabolites. J. nat. Cancer Inst., 41, 985-1036

Kaney, A.R. & Atwood, K.C. (1964) Radiomimetic action of polyimine chemisterilants in *Neurospora*. Nature (Lond.), 201, 1006-1008

LaBrecque, G.C. (1961) Studies with three alkylating agents as house fly sterilants. J. econ. Entomol., 54, 684-689

Manna, G.K. & Das, P.K. (1973) Effect of two chemosterilants apholate and hempa on the bone-marrow chromosomes of mice. Canad. J. Genet. Cytol., 15, 451-459

Ottmann, G., Agahigian, H., Hooks, H., Vickers, G.D., Kober, E. & Rätz, R. (1964) (1-Aziridinyl)cyclotriphosphaza-1,3,5-trienes. Inorg. Chem., 3, 753-757

Rätz, R.F.W. & Grundmann, C.J. (1958) US Patent 2,858,306, 28 October, Olin Mathieson Chemical Corporation

Rätz, R., Kober, E., Grundmann, C. & Ottmann, G. (1964) Syntheses and reactions of 2,2,4,4,6,6-hexakis(1-aziridinyl)cyclotriphosphaza-1,3,5-triene and related compounds. Inorg. Chem., 3, 757-761

Smith, C.N., LaBrecque, G.C. & Borkovec, A.B. (1964) Insect chemosterilants. In: Smith, R.F. & Mittler, T.E., eds, Annual Review of Entomology, Vol. 9, Palo Alto, California, Annual Reviews Inc., pp. 269-284

Stecher, P.G., ed. (1968) The Merck Index, 8th ed., Rahway, N.J., Merck & Co., p. 94

AZIRIDINE

1. Chemical and Physical Data

1.1 Synonyms and trade names

Chem. Abstr. Reg. Serial No.:   151-56-4

Chem. Abstr. Name: Aziridine

Azacyclopropane; dihydro-1H-azirine; dimethylenimine; EI; ethylene imine; ethyleneimine; ethylenimine; ethylimine

1.2 Chemical formula and molecular weight

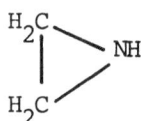

$$\begin{array}{c} H_2C \\ | \quad\quad NH \\ H_2C \end{array}$$
C_2H_5N Mol. wt: 43.1

1.3 Chemical and physical properties of the pure substance

(a) Description: Colourless liquid with intense ammoniacal odour; fumes in air;   flammable

(b) Boiling-point: 56-57°C at 760 mm Hg

(c) Melting-point: -73.96°C

(d) Density: d_4^{24} 0.832

(e) Refractive index: n_D^{25} 1.412

(f) Spectroscopy data: Extensive data have been compiled by Dermer & Ham (1969).

(g) Identity and purity test: Forms picrate yellow needles (m.p., 142°C; crystallized from water);   forms oxalate needles (m.p., 115°C; decomposition)

(h) Solubility: Miscible with water and virtually all organic solvents

(i) Volatility: Vapour pressure is 160 mm Hg at 20°C.

(j) Stability: Hydrolyses in aqueous solutions to give ethanolamine

1.4 Technical products and impurities

Aziridine is available commercially in bottles, in 5-, 25- and 55-gallon steel cylinders and in tank cars (Dow Chemical Company, 1966). Specifications for commercial aziridine require: 99 mole % minimum active ingredient, 50-150 mg/l sodium, 0.2% by weight maximum water, and 0.2% by weight maximum non-volatile matter (Dermer & Hart, 1966).

2. Production, Use, Occurrence and Analysis

For important background information on this section, see preamble, p. 17.

A review on aziridine has been published (Dermer & Ham, 1969).

2.1 Production and use

Aziridine was prepared by the dehydrobromination of 2-bromoethylamine by Gabriel in 1888. Commercial production by the cyclization of 2-aminoethyl hydrogen sulphate began in Germany in 1938. In 1963, a US company announced (and probably began on a commercial basis) production of aziridine by the reaction of ammonia and ethylene dichloride (Dermer & Hart, 1966).

Four US producers manufactured 680,000 kg of this chemical in 1964 (Dermer & Hart, 1966). It was listed by one manufacturer in annual US Tariff Commission production reports over a consecutive four-year period, appearing last in 1968 (US Tariff Commission, 1970). Currently there is only one US manufacturer, with an estimated annual production of less than 2.2 million kg.

Aziridine is produced in Europe; however, one producer in the Federal Republic of Germany suspended sales of this chemical and all derivatives except polyethyleneimine in 1973. This action was apparently taken as a result of the US Occupational Safety and Health Administration's inclusion of aziridine on a list of "occupational carcinogens". Several hundred thousand kg per year of polyethyleneimine are presently sold to the paper industry; thus, small quantities of aziridine are consumed captively in the manufacture of its derivatives.

Aziridine has been produced commercially in Japan since 1964. Production during the period 1970-1974 is estimated to have been 600,000 kg per year; there is currently only one producer.

Approximately 50% of the aziridine produced in the US is polymerized to polyethyleneimine containing less than 1 mg/kg residual monomer. Principal uses for polyethyleneimine are as a flocculant in water treatment and in the textile and paper industries where it is used as a wet-strength additive, since its cationic nature results in adhesion to cellulose compounds (Dow Chemical Company, 1966). It has also been used as an adhesion promoter in various coating applications and as an intermediate in drug, cosmetic and dye manufacture.

Aziridine is also believed to be used in the production of 2-aziridinyl ethanol and of triethylenemelamine (Stecher, 1968) and as an intermediate and monomer for oil additive compounds, ion exchange resins, coating resins, pharmaceuticals, adhesives, polymer stabilizers and surfactants (Hawley, 1971).

In Japan, aziridine is believed to be used principally in the production of polyethyleneimine, although it is also used to produce taurine and as an intermediate in the production of pesticides and dyestuffs.

2.2 Occurrence

Aziridine is not known to occur in nature.

In the US, occupational exposure is subject to Occupational Safety and Health Administration standards. These call for monitoring, control methods, medical surveillance, records and reports and require that an employee's exposure to aziridine during a 40-hour week not exceed an 8-hour time-weighted average of 1 mg/m^3 (0.5 ppm) (US Code of Federal Regulations, 1973).

In the Federal Republic of Germany and the German Democratic Republic maximum exposure to aziridine is limited to 1 mg/m^3 (0.5 ppm), and in the USSR to 0.02 mg/m^3 (Winell, 1975).

2.3 Analysis

Several methods of analysis have been described, including colorimetric estimation in non-aqueous medium and in aqueous solution (<5 µg/ml) by reaction with 4-(4'-nitrobenzyl)pyridine (Epstein *et al.*, 1955; Preussmann *et al.*, 1969) and in air samples (5-10 ppm v/v) (Crompton, 1965; Salyamon & Popelkovskaya, 1972); and chromatography on silica gel plates (Sawicki & Sawicki, 1969) and on paper (Fishbein & Cavanaugh, 1965). An automated colorimetric method (Terranova, 1969), a chromatographic separation on ion-exchange resins (Shimamura *et al.*, 1973) and a gas chromatographic method (Di Lorenzo & Russo, 1968) have also been reported.

3. Biological Data Relevant to the Evaluation of Carcinogenic Risk to Man

3.1 Carcinogenicity and related studies in animals

(a) Oral administration

Mouse: Two groups of 18 male and 18 female mice of the (C57Bl/6x C3H/Anf)F_1 or (C57Bl/6xAKR)F_1 strain were given the same absolute amount of 4.64 mg/kg bw aziridine by stomach tube daily from the 7th to 28th day of age. Subsequently, the substance was fed at a concentration of 13 mg/kg of diet throughout the observation period of 77 or 78 weeks. The total numbers of mice with tumours were 16/17 males (15 with hepatomas, 15 with pulmonary tumours) and 15/15 females (11 with hepatomas, 15 with pulmonary tumours) of the (C57Bl/6xC3H/Anf)F_1 strain; 16/16 males (9 with hepatomas, 12 with pulmonary tumours) and 11/11 females (2 with hepatomas, 10 with pulmonary tumours, 2 with lymphomas) of the (C57Bl/6xAKR)F_1 strain. The number of hepatomas and pulmonary tumours combined was significantly greater than that in controls (P=0.01) for all 4 groups of mice. The incidences of hepatomas in male and female controls of the two strains were 8/79 and 0/87 in (C57Bl/6xC3H/Anf)F_1 mice and 5/90 and 1/82 in (C57Bl/6x AKR)F_1 mice. The respective incidences of lung tumours were 5/79, 3/87, 10/90 and 3/82 (Innes *et al.*, 1969; National Technical Information Service, 1968).

(b) Subcutaneous and/or intramuscular administration

Suckling mouse: In groups of 18 male and 18 female (C57Bl/6xC3H/Anf)F_1 mice and 18 male and 18 female (C57Bl/6xAKR)F_1 mice given single s.c.

40

injections of 4.64 mg/kg bw aziridine on the 7th day of age followed by observation up to 80 weeks, tumours developed in 7/18 males (2 lymphomas, 2 hepatomas, 5 pulmonary tumours) of the (C57Bl/6xC3H/Anf)F$_1$ strain and in 6/18 males (6 lung tumours) of the (C57Bl/6xAKR)F$_1$ strain. One female of each strain developed a lung tumour. The total number of tumours in males of both strains was significantly greater than that in controls (P=0.01) (National Technical Information Service, 1968).

Rat: A group of 6 male and 6 female stock albino rats, 80-120 g, was given twice weekly s.c. injections of aziridine dissolved in arachis oil (total dose, 20 mg/kg bw administered over 67 injections). Five males and 1 female developed sarcomas at the injection site within 355-511 days. Of 19 control rats treated with arachis oil, 1/10 males developed a sarcoma at the injection site (568th day) and 1/9 females developed a fibroma at the injection site (643rd day) [P<0.05]. Fourteen controls died between 209-676 days. An additional group of 6 male and 6 female rats received twice weekly s.c. injections of aziridine in water (total doses, 12 and 10 mg/kg bw in males and females, given over 59 injections). One male developed a tumour described as a transitional-cell carcinoma in the kidney (456th day) and 2 females developed sarcomas at the injection site (166th and 447th days) (Walpole et al., 1954).

3.2 Other relevant biological data

Aziridine is toxic to mice, the LC$_{50}$ being 3.93 mg/l (observation time, 10 days) for animals exposed for 10 minutes (Silver & McGrath, 1948), and to rats and guinea-pigs, the latter being more sensitive. The LC$_{50}$ after 3 hours in rats and guinea-pigs was about 250 mg/l in air; exposure to 25 mg/l caused deaths within 4-8 hours due to lung injury and necrosis of kidney tubular epithelium (Carpenter et al., 1948). The oral LD$_{50}$ was 15 mg/kg bw in male albino rats (Smyth et al., 1941) and the LD$_{50}$ by skin contact was 14 mg/kg bw in guinea-pigs (Carpenter et al., 1948). Changes in blood vessels, destruction of lymphatic follicles, necrosis of spermato-genic epithelium, degeneration in the liver, kidneys and myocardium and extracapillary glomerulonephritis have been observed. Daily inhalation in air of 0.01 mg/l for 4 hours for 1.5 months caused catarrhal bronchitis, diminishing of lymphatic elements in lymph glands and degenerative changes in liver and kidneys in rats (Zaeva et al., 1966).

About half of 0.30-0.42 mg/kg bw ^{14}C-aziridine administered intraperitoneally to rats was excreted in the urine. A small amount of aziridine was excreted as such in the urine, but the major portion of the excreted radioactivity was found as a number of unidentified products. Three to five percent of the activity was expired as CO_2, and 1-3% was expired probably as aziridine. Radioactivity was widely distributed, with some accumulation in the liver, intestines, caecum, spleen and kidneys (Wright & Rowe, 1967).

In *Neurospora crassa*, aziridine produced leaky mutants, mutants with non-polarized complementation patterns, mutants with polarized complementation patterns, non-complementing mutants and multilocus deletions (Ong & de Serres, 1973). In *Saccharomyces cerevisiae*, it induced mitotic recombination (Zimmermann & von Laer, 1967) and gene conversion (Zimmermann, 1971).

In *Drosophila melanogaster* it induces both transmissible translocations and sex-linked recessive lethals (Alexander & Glanges, 1965; Srám, 1970), and it causes specific locus mutations in silkworms (*Bombyx mori*) (Inagaki & Oster, 1969).

In barley aziridine induces a high frequency of chlorophyll-deficient mutations (Nawar et al., 1971) and a wide distribution of *eceriferum* mutations (von Wettstein et al., 1968).

When rabbits were inseminated with spermatozoa which had been treated with aziridine *in vitro*, only 40% of embryos were viable relative to the number of *corpora lutea*, in comparison to 78% in controls (Nuzhdin & Nizhnik, 1968).

Acute toxic effects of inhaled aziridine vapours in man were first reported by Danehy & Pflaum (1938). Cases of accidental exposure to aziridine and N-ethyl aziridine vapours involving a febrile or afebrile reaction, conjunctivitis, respiratory tract irritation, oedema and albuminuria have also been reported (Weightman & Hoyle, 1964). Aziridine also causes burns on the skin.

3.3 Observations in man

No data were available to the Working Group.

4. Comments on Data Reported and Evaluation[1]

4.1 Animal data

Aziridine is carcinogenic in two strains of mice following its oral administration, producing an increased incidence of liver-cell and pulmonary tumours. Subcutaneous injection of single doses in suckling mice produced an increased incidence of lung tumours in males. In one experiment in rats it increased the incidence of tumours at the injection site following its subcutaneous injection in oil.

4.2 Human data

No case reports or epidemiological studies were available to the Working Group.

---

[1]See also the section, "Animal Data in Relation to the Evaluation of Risk to Man" in the introduction to this volume, p. 15.

5. References

Alexander, M.L. & Glanges, E. (1965) Genetic damage induced by ethylene-imine. Proc. nat. Acad. Sci. (Wash.), 53, 282-288

Carpenter, C.P., Smyth, H.F. & Shaffer, C.B. (1948) The acute toxicity of ethyleneimine to small animals. J. industr. Hyg. Toxicol., 30, 2-6

Crompton, T.R. (1965) Determination of traces of ethyleneimine monomer in samples of air. Analyst, 90, 107-111

Danehy, J.P. & Pflaum, D.J. (1938) Toxicity of ethylene imine. Industr. Eng. Chem., 30, 778

Dermer, O.C. & Ham, G.E. (1969) Ethyleneimine and other Aziridines: Chemistry and Applications, New York, Academic Press

Dermer, O.C. & Hart, A.W. (1966) Imines, Cyclic. In: Kirk, R.E. & Othmer, D.F., eds, Encyclopedia of Chemical Technology, 2nd ed., Vol. 11, New York, John Wiley & Sons, pp. 526-548

Di Lorenzo, A. & Russo, G. (1968) Gas chromatographic analysis of aliphatic amines and imines. J. Gas Chromat., 6, 509-512

Dow Chemical Company (1966) Ethylenimine: Chemistry, Handling, Uses, Midland, Michigan

Epstein, J., Rosenthal, R.W. & Ess, R.J. (1955) Use of γ-(4-nitrobenzyl)-pyridine as analytical reagent for ethylenimines and alkylating agents. Analyt. Chem., 27, 1435-1439

Fishbein, L. & Cavanaugh, M.A. (1965) Detection and paper chromatography of N-substituted hydroxy-, 2-hydroxyethyl-, 2-chloroethyl- and N,N-bis-(2-hydroxyethyl)-derivatives. J. Chromat., 20, 283-294

Hawley, G.G. (1971) The Condensed Chemical Dictionary, 8th ed., New York, Van Nostrand Reinhold, p. 367

Inagaki, E. & Oster, I.I. (1969) Changes in the mutational response of silkworm spermatozoa exposed to mono- and polyfunctional alkylating agents following storage. Mutation Res., 7, 425-432

Innes, J.R.M., Ulland, B.M., Valerio, M.G., Petrucelli, L., Fishbein, L., Hart, E.R., Pallotta, A.J., Bates, R.R., Falk, H.L., Gart, J.J., Klein, M., Mitchell, I. & Peters, J. (1969) Bioassay of pesticides and industrial chemicals for tumorigenicity in mice: a preliminary note. J. nat. Cancer Inst., 42, 1101-1114

National Technical Information Service (1968) Evaluation of Carcinogenic, Teratogenic and Mutagenic Activities of Selected Pesticides and Industrial Chemicals, Vol. 1, Carcinogenic Study, Washington DC, US Department of Commerce

Nawar, M.M., Konzak, C.F. & Nilan, R.A. (1971) Comparative studies of the biological effectiveness of nitrogen mustards, ethyleneimine and γ-rays. Mutation Res., 11, 339-346

Nuzhdin, N.I. & Nizhnik, G.V. (1968) Fertilization and embryonic development of rabbits after treatment of spermatozoa in vitro with chemical mutagens. Dokl. Akad. Nauk SSSR, Otd. Biol., 181, 419-422

Ong, T.-M. & de Serres, F.J. (1973) Mutagenic activity of ethylenimine in Neurospora crassa. Mutation Res., 18, 251-258

Preussmann, R., Schneider, H. & Epple, F. (1969) Untersuchungen zum Nachweis alkylierender Agentien. II. Der Nachweis verschiedener Klassen alkylierender Agentien mit einer Modifikation der Farbreaktion mit 4-(4-Nitrobenzyl)pyridin (NBP). Arzneimittel-Forsch., 19, 1059-1073

Salyamon, G.S. & Popelkovskaya, M.V. (1972) Determination of ethylenimine in the air. Gig. i Sanit., 37, 117-118

Sawicki, E. & Sawicki, C.R. (1969) Analysis of alkylating agents: applications to air pollution. Ann. N.Y. Acad. Sci., 163, 895-920

Shimomura, K., Hsu, T-J. & Walton, H.F. (1973) Ligand-exchange chromatography of aziridines and ethanolamines. Analyt. Chem., 45, 501-505

Silver, S.D. & McGrath, F.P. (1948) A comparison of acute toxicities of ethylene imine and ammonia to mice. J. industr. Hyg. Toxicol., 30, 7-9

Smyth, H.F., Jr, Seaton, J. & Fischer, L. (1941) The single dose toxicity of some glycols and derivatives. J. industr. Hyg. Toxicol., 23, 259-268

Srám, R.J. (1970) The effect of storage on the frequency of translocations in Drosophila melanogaster. Mutation Res., 9, 243-244

Stecher, P.G., ed. (1968) The Merck Index, 8th ed., Rahway, N.J., Merck & Co., p. 435

Terranova, A.C. (1969) Automated procedure for the determination of the aziridine moieties of N,N'-tetramethylenebis(1-aziridinecarboxamide) and other compounds containing aziridine. J. agric. Fd Chem., 17, 1047-1051

US Code of Federal Regulations (1973) Occupational Safety and Health Standards, Title 29, part 1910.93, Washington DC, US Government Printing Office, p. 21

US Tariff Commission (1970) Synthetic Organic Chemicals, US Production and Sales, 1968, TC Publication 327, Washington DC, US Government Printing Office, p. 41

Walpole, A.L., Roberts, D.C., Rose, F.L., Hendry, J.A. & Homer, R.F. (1954) Cytotoxic agents. IV. The carcinogenic actions of some monofunctional ethyleneimine derivatives. Brit. J. Pharmacol., 9, 306-323

Weightman, J. & Hoyle, J.P. (1964) Accidental exposure to ethylenimine and N-ethyl-ethylenimine vapors. J. Amer. med. Ass., 189, 543-545

von Wettstein, D., Lundovist, U. & von Wettstein-Knowles, P. (1968) The mutagen specificities of 44 eceriferum loci in barley. In: Mutations in Plant Breeding, vol. 2, Panel Proc. Series, Int. Atomic Energy Agency, New York, Unipub., pp. 273-275

Winell, M. (1975) An international comparison of hygienic standards for chemicals in the work environment. Ambio, 4, 34-36

Wright, G.J. & Rowe, V.K. (1967) Ethylenimine: studies of the distribution and metabolism in the rat using carbon-14. Toxicol. appl. Pharmacol., 11, 575-584

Zaeva, G.N., Timofievskaya, L.A., Fedorova, V.I., Ivanov, V.N. & Vinogradova, E.L. (1966) An evaluation of acute and subacute toxicity of ethylenimine. Toksikol. Novykh Prom. Khim. Veshchestv, 8, 41-60

Zimmermann, F.K. (1971) Induction of mitotic gene conversion by mutagens. Mutation Res., 11, 327-337

Zimmermann, F.K. & von Laer, U. (1967) Induction of mitotic recombination with ethyleneimine in Saccharomyces cerevisiae. Mutation Res., 4, 377-379

2-(1-AZIRIDINYL)ETHANOL

1. Chemical and Physical Data

1.1 Synonyms and trade names

Chem. Abstr. Reg. Serial No.:   1072-52-2

Chem. Abstr. Name: 1-Aziridineethanol

β-Hydroxy-1-ethylaziridine;   *N*-(β-hydroxyethyl)aziridine;   *N*-(2-hydroxyethyl)aziridine;   *N*-(2-hydroxyethyl)ethylenimine;   2-(hydroxy-ethyl)ethylenimine;   1-(2-hydroxyethyl)ethylenimine

1.2 Chemical formula and molecular weight

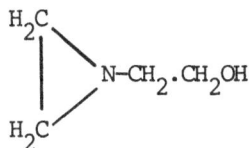

$$\begin{array}{c} H_2C \\ | \\ H_2C \end{array} \!\!\!\! > N\!-\!CH_2.CH_2OH$$

C_4H_9NO Mol. wt: 87.1

1.3 Chemical and physical properties of the pure substance

(a) Description: Colourless liquid

(b) Boiling-point: 40-45°C at 1.9-2.5 mm Hg;   69-71°C at 16 mm Hg; 154-156°C at 760 mm Hg

(c) Refractive index: n_D^{25} 1.453; n_D^{26} 1.447

(d) Reactivity: Hydrolyses to give diethanolamine

1.4 Technical products and impurities

No data were available to the Working Group.

2. Production, Use, Occurrence and Analysis

For important background information on this section, see preamble, p. 17.

2.1 Production and use

2-(1-Aziridinyl)ethanol can be prepared by the addition of aziridine to ethylene oxide (Wilson, 1949). According to industry sources, it has been produced commercially, only in the US, since about 1965. Production by one company in 1973 was about 45,000 kg.

2-(1-Aziridinyl)ethanol is reported to be used commercially in the US in the modification of latex polymers for coatings, textile resins and starches. It is also used by manufacturers of modified cellulose products such as paper, wood fibres and fabrics.

It has been tested as an insect chemosterilant (Borkovec *et al.*, 1968), but it is not used commercially for this purpose because of problems associated with its application to insects, its toxicity and environmental effects.

2.2 Occurrence

2-(1-Aziridinyl)ethanol is not known to occur in nature.

2.3 Analysis

Chromatographic separation on ion-exchange resins (Shimomura *et al.*, 1973) and its determination by gas-liquid chromatography (Zager *et al.*, 1969) have been described.

3. Biological Data Relevant to the Evaluation of Carcinogenic Risk to Man

3.1 Carcinogenicity and related studies in animals

Subcutaneous and/or intramuscular administration

Mouse: Thirty 6-8-week old female ICR/Ha Swiss mice were given weekly s.c. injections of 0.3 mg 2-(1-aziridinyl)ethanol in 0.05 ml tricaprylin for 75 weeks, the duration of the experiment. After 21 weeks, when the first tumour occurred, 26 mice were alive and 10 mice had developed tumours at the injection site described as lymphosarcomas (5), fibrosarcomas (4) and an adenosarcoma (1). No tumours at the injection site occurred in 30 control mice treated with the vehicle for up to 93 weeks (Van Duuren *et al.*, 1971).

3.2 Other relevant biological data

Single doses of 40-50 mg/kg bw 2-(1-aziridinyl)ethanol given intravenously to cats caused death in some animals within 2-4 hours (Zager *et al.*, 1969).

Single oral doses ranging from 125-1000 mg/kg bw produced liver necrosis in rats. Oral administration of 10 mg/kg bw to rats for 5 days caused depletion of the bone marrow and atrophy of the lymph nodes, thymus and spleen (Zager *et al.*, 1969).

2-(1-Aziridinyl)ethanol induced sex-linked recessive lethals in *Drosophila melanogaster* (Filippova *et al.*, 1967).

3.3 Observations in man

No data were available to the Working Group.

4. Comments on Data Reported and Evaluation[1]

4.1 Animal data

2-(1-Aziridinyl)ethanol is carcinogenic in mice, producing malignant tumours at the site of its subcutaneous injection in the only available study.

4.2 Human data

No case reports or epidemiological studies were available to the Working Group.

---

[1]See also the section, "Animal Data in Relation to the Evaluation of Risk to Man" in the introduction to this volume, p. 15.

5. References

Borkovec, A.B., Fye, R.L. & LaBrecque, G.C. (1968) Aziridinyl chemosterilants for houseflies, ARS 33-129, Washington DC, US Department
of Agriculture

Filippova, L.M., Pan'shin, O.A. & Kostyankovskii, R.G. (1967) Chemical
mutagens. IV. Mutagenic activity of germinal systems. Genetika,
3, 134-148 WTable 3, compound no. 5X

Shimomura, K., Hsu, T.-J. & Walton, H.F. (1973) Ligand-exchange chromatography of aziridines and ethanolamines. Analyt. Chem., 45, 501-505

Van Duuren, B.L., Melchionne, S., Blair, R., Goldschmidt, B.M. & Katz, C.
(1971) Carcinogenicity of isosters of epoxides and lactones:
aziridine ethanol, propane sultone and related compounds. J. nat.
Cancer Inst., 46, 143-149

Wilson, A.L. (1949) Hydroxyalkyl alkylenimines. US Patent, 2,475,068,
July 5, Carbide and Carbon Chemicals Corp.

Zager, R.F., McCarty, L.P. & Standaert, F.G. (1969) The pharmacology of
2-aziridinyl ethanol. J. Pharmacol. exp. Ther., 166, 205-216

AZIRIDYL BENZOQUINONE

1. Chemical and Physical Data

1.1 Synonyms and trade names

Chem. Abstr. Reg. Serial No.: 800-24-8

Chem. Abstr. Name: 2,5-Bis(1-aziridinyl)-3,6-bis(2-methoxyethoxy)-*para*-benzoquinone

Benzoquinone aziridine; 2,5-bis(1-aziridinyl)-3,6-bis(2-methoxy-ethoxy)-2,5-cyclohexadiene-1,4-dione; 2,5-bisaziridinyl-3,6-bis-(methoxyethoxy)quinone; 2,5-bisaziridinyl-3,6-bis(2-methoxyethoxy)-quinone; 2,5-bismethoxyethoxy-3,6-bisethyleneimino-1,4-benzoquinone; 3,6-bis(β-methoxyethoxy)-2,5-bis(ethylenimino)-*para*-benzoquinone; 2,5-methoxyethoxy-3,6-bis(ethylenimino)-1,4-benzoquinone

A 139; Bay A 139; Bayer A 139; Bayer E 39; Bayer E 39 Soluble; E 39 Soluble

1.2 Chemical formula and molecular weight

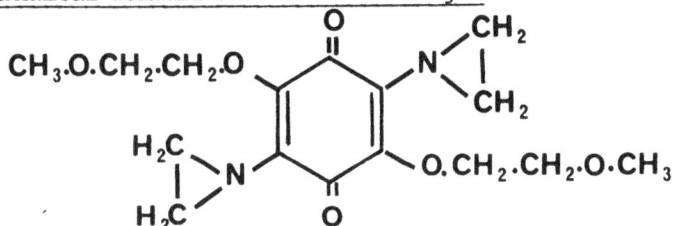

$C_{16}H_{22}N_2O_6$

Mol. wt: 338.3

1.3 Chemical and physical properties of the pure substance

(a) Description: Grey needles from petroleum ether

(b) Melting-point: 79-80.5°C

(c) Stability: Unstable in water or polar solvents

1.4 Technical products and impurities

No data were available to the Working Group.

2. Production, Use, Occurrence and Analysis

For important background information on this section, see preamble, p. 17.

2.1 Production and use

Aziridyl benzoquinone can be prepared by the addition of 3,6-dichloro-2,5-di(1-aziridinyl)-1,4-benzoquinone to the sodium salt of ethylene glycol monomethyl ether (Farbenfabriken Bayer AG, 1958). It has been produced for research purposes only; however, it has reportedly been used clinically for the treatment of human cancer (Anon., 1959).

This chemical has also been tested as an insect chemosterilant (Crystal & LaChance, 1963), but it is believed that problems associated with its application to insects, its toxicity and possible environmental effects have prevented its use in this way on a commercial basis.

2.2 Occurrence

Aziridyl benzoquinone is not known to occur in nature.

2.3 Analysis

An automated colorimetric method using 4-(4'-nitrobenzyl)pyridine for the determination of a number of aziridine compounds has been proposed (Terranova, 1969).

3. Biological Data Relevant to the Evaluation of Carcinogenic Risk to Man

3.1 Carcinogenicity and related studies in animals

Intraperitoneal administration

Mouse: Four groups each of 15 male and 15 female 4-6 week old A/J mice were injected with 0.2 ml of an aqueous solution of aziridyl benzoquinone 3 times per week for 4 weeks (total doses, 0.47, 1.87, 7.5 and 30 mg/kg bw). The experiment was terminated at 39 weeks and lung tumours were found in 18/29 (62%), 8/22 (36%), 16/25 (64%) and 24/28 (86%) treated mice, compared with 39.5% and 31.4% of 385 male and 392 female vehicle-injected controls. The numbers of lung tumours per mouse were 0.50 and 0.36

in male and female controls, compared with 0.8, 0.4, 1.4 and 2.9 in the four treated groups. In these experiments aziridyl benzoquinone was reported to be about 12 times less potent than uracil mustard on a molar basis (Shimkin *et al.*, 1966). [Tumour incidences were significantly different from those in controls (P<0.01) at the lowest and two highest dose levels.]

3.2 Other relevant biological data

Aziridyl benzoquinone induced a high frequency of chromosome aberrations in freshly-prepared cultures of human leucocytes (Beek & Obe, 1974; Obe, 1973).

3.3 Observations in man

No data were available to the Working Group.

4. Comments on Data Reported and Evaluation[1]

4.1 Animal data

Aziridyl benzoquinone is carcinogenic in mice following its intraperitoneal injection, the only species and route tested, producing an increase in the incidence of lung tumours.

4.2 Human data

No case reports or epidemiological studies were available to the Working Group.

---

[1]See also the section, "Animal Data in Relation to the Evaluation of Risk to Man" in the introduction to this volume, p. 15.

5. References

Anon. (1959) Cancer. Chemical and Engineering News, October 12, pp. 53-71

Beek, B. & Obe, G. (1974) The human leukocyte test system. II. Different
    sensitivities of sub-populations to a chemical mutagen. Mutation Res.,
    24, 395-398

Crystal, M.M. & LaChance, L.E. (1963) Modification of reproduction in
    insects treated with alkylating agents. I. Inhibition of ovarian
    growth and egg production and hatchability. Biol. Bull., 125, 270-279

Farbenfabriken Bayer AG (1958) Substituted 1-aziridinylquinones. British
    Patent, 793,707, April 23

Obe, G. (1973) Chromosome breaking activity of A139 in human lymphocytes
    in vitro. Experientia, 29, 1154-1155

Shimkin, M.B., Weisburger, J.H., Weisburger, E.K., Gubareff, N. &
    Suntzeff, V. (1966) Bioassay of 29 alkylating chemicals by the pulmonary-
    tumor response in strain A mice. J. nat. Cancer Inst., 36, 915-935

Terranova, A.C. (1969) Automated procedure for the determination of the
    aziridine moieties of N,N'-tetramethylenebis(1-aziridinecarboxamide)
    and other compounds containing aziridine. J. agric. Fd Chem., 17,
    1047-1051

BIS(1-AZIRIDINYL)MORPHOLINOPHOSPHINE SULPHIDE

1. Chemical and Physical Data

1.1 Synonyms and trade names

Chem. Abstr. Reg. Serial No.:   2168-68-5

Chem. Abstr. Name: 4-[Bis(1-aziridinyl)phosphinothioyl]morpholine

N,N'-Diethylenemorpholinophosphinothioic diamide;   *N,N'*-diethylene-
N'-(3-oxapentamethylene)phosphorothioic triamide;   diethylene oxapenta-
methylenethiophosphoramide;   morzid;   opspa;   *N*-(3-oxapentamethylene)-
N',N"-diethylenethiophosphoramide;   thiomorpholidophosphoric diethylen-
imide

1.2 Chemical formula and molecular weight

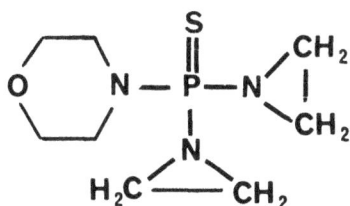

$C_8H_{16}N_3OPS$

Mol. wt: 233.2

1.3 Chemical and physical properties of the pure substance

(a) <u>Description</u>:   White crystals

(b) <u>Melting-point</u>:   75-77°C

(c) <u>Solubility</u>:   Slightly soluble in water;   very soluble in benzene,
toluene and hot petroleum ether

(d) <u>Reactivity</u>:   Boiling for 1 hour in 1 N HCl leads to a quantitative
release of morpholine with a yield of phosphate limited to 10%,
which indicates that the morpholine side chain is released much
more readily than are the aziridine rings (Maller & Heidelberger,
1957b).

1.4 Technical products and impurities

No data were available to the Working Group.

2. Production, Use, Occurrence and Analysis

For important background information on this section, see preamble, p. 17.

2.1 Production and use

Bis(1-aziridinyl)morpholinophosphine sulphide (opspa) can be prepared by the reaction of morpholine with $PSCl_3$ in the presence of triethylamine, followed by reaction of the product [N-(3-oxapentamethylene)-N',N''-dichloro-thiophosphoric acid] with aziridine in the presence of triethylamine (Parker et al., 1952).

Opspa has been produced for research purposes and has been tested clinically as an antineoplastic agent (Anon., 1959). It has also been shown to be effective as an insect chemosterilant (Klasen et al., 1968; LaBrecque, 1961; Smith et al., 1964), but it is believed that problems associated with its application to insects, its toxicity and possible environmental effects have prevented its use in this way on a commercial basis.

2.2 Occurrence

Opspa is not known to occur in nature.

2.3 Analysis

The standard titration method for the determination of intact aziridine rings can be used for estimation of this chemical (Heidelberger & Baumann, 1957). For determinations in biological fluids, the procedure for the estimation of alkylating agents based on a colour reaction with 4-(4'-nitrobenzyl)pyridine could be used (Truhaut et al., 1963). With this method the limit of detection is less than 1 µg/ml (Terranova, 1969).

3. Biological Data Relevant to the Evaluation of Carcinogenic Risk to Man

3.1 Carcinogenicity and related studies in animals

Intraperitoneal administration

Mouse: Four groups each of 15 male and 15 female 4-6 week old A/J

mice were injected with opspa dissolved in water 3 times per week for 4
weeks; animals were killed 39 weeks after the first injection (total
doses, 1.9, 7.5, 30 and 120 mg/kg bw). The numbers of surviving animals
at that time were 28, 28, 30 and 24; and 11 (39%), 16 (57%), 13 (43%) and
20 (83%) of these had developed tumours, the average numbers of lung tumours
per mouse being 0.4, 1.0, 0.6 and 2.0. In 385 male and 392 female vehicle-
injected controls, 39.5% of males and 31.4% of females developed lung
tumours, with averages of 0.50 and 0.36 lung tumours per mouse. In these
experiments opspa was reported to be 125 times less potent than uracil
mustard (Shimkin *et al.*, 1966). [Tumour incidences were significantly
different from those in controls at the highest dose level ($P<0.001$) and
at the 7.5 mg/kg bw dose level ($P<0.02$).]

3.2 Other relevant biological data

Acute toxicities for different species have been reported; monkeys,
dogs and rats were more sensitive to the drug than mice (Schmidt *et al.*,
1965a,b).

In mice treated with ^{14}C- or ^{32}P-labelled opspa, the compound was
metabolized by desulphuration to the corresponding phosphoramide, bis(1-
aziridinyl)morpholinophosphine oxide; and some was converted to morpholine
and to inorganic phosphate (Maller & Heidelberger, 1957b). The principal
excretion route was *via* the urine, in which 50-75% of the radioactivity
appeared during the first 24 hours; only small amounts were expired as
carbon dioxide or voided with the faeces (Maller & Heidelberger, 1957a).
Twice as much morpholine was excreted in the urine after oral as compared
to i.p. administration of opspa (Heidelberger & Baumann, 1957; Maller &
Heidelberger, 1957b). In rats, unchanged opspa was found in trace amounts
only in urine and tumour tissue (Maller & Heidelberger, 1957b).

Administration of compound SKF 525A (β-diethylaminoethyldiphenyl-
propylacetate) to rats prior to an injection of opspa inhibited its degradation; thus, increased amounts of unchanged drug appeared in the urine,
plasma and liver (Maller & Heidelberger, 1957b).

In rats there was no evidence of selective localization in normal
or in transplantable tumour tissues. Tissue fractionation studies

demonstrated that the major part of the radioactivity present in liver and tumour tissue was in the aqueous and lipid fractions; some material was bound to proteins, and small quantities were found in the crude nucleic acid fraction (Maller & Heidelberger, 1957a).

In man, absorption of ^{32}P-opspa from the site of its i.m. injection was very much faster from a saline vehicle than from a corn oil vehicle. Excretion was principally *via* the urine: after 3 days about 50% of the injected radioactivity was recovered in the urine, and only trace quantities were excreted in the faeces. As in the rat, there was no evidence of selective localization in normal tissues or in tumour biopsy samples (Maller *et al.*, 1957).

3.3 Observations in man

No data were available to the Working Group.

4. Comments on Data Reported and Evaluation[1]

4.1 Animal data

Bis(1-aziridinyl)morpholinophosphine sulphide is carcinogenic in mice following its intraperitoneal injection, the only species and route tested, producing an increase in the incidence of lung tumours.

4.2 Human data

No case reports or epidemiological studies were available to the Working Group.

---

[1]See also the section, "Animal Data in Relation to the Evaluation of Risk to Man" in the introduction to this volume, p. 15.

5. References

Anon. (1959) Cancer. Chemical and Engineering News, October 12, pp. 53-71

Heidelberger, C. & Baumann, M.E. (1957) Studies on opspa. I. The effect of several phosphoramides on transplanted tumors. Cancer Res., 17, 277-283

Klasen, W., Norland, J.F. & Borkovec, A.B. (1968) Potential chemosterilants for boll weevils. J. econ. Entomol., 61, 401-407

LaBrecque, G.C. (1961) Studies with three alkylating agents as house fly sterilants. J. econ. Entomol., 54, 684-689

Maller, R.K. & Heidelberger, C. (1957a) Studies on opspa. II. Distribution and excretion of radioactivity following administration of opspa-C^{14} and opspa-P^{32} to the rat. Cancer Res., 17, 284-290

Maller, R.K. & Heidelberger, C. (1957b) Studies on opspa. IV. Metabolism in the rat and human. Cancer Res., 17, 296-301

Maller, R.K., McIver, F.A. & Heidelberger, C. (1957) Studies on opspa. III. Distribution and excretion of radioactivity following administration of opspa-C^{14} and opspa-P^{32} to humans. Cancer Res., 17, 291-295

Parker, R.P., Seeger, D.R. & Kuh, E. (1952) Phosphoric acid ethylene amides. US Patent, 2,606,900, August 12

Schmidt, L.H., Fradkin, R., Sullivan, R. & Flowers, A. (1965a) Comparative pharmacology of alkylating agents. I. Toxicity data on rats and mice. Cancer Chemother. Rep., Suppl. 2, 1-401

Schmidt, L.H., Fradkin, R., Sullivan, R. & Flowers, A. (1965b) Comparative pharmacology of alkylating agents. III. Toxicity data on monkeys and dogs. Cancer Chemother. Rep., Suppl. 2, 1017-1528

Shimkin, M.B., Weisburger, J.H., Weisburger, E.K., Gubareff, N. & Suntzeff, V. (1966) Bioassay of 29 alkylating chemicals by the pulmonary-tumor response in strain A mice. J. nat. Cancer Inst., 36, 915-935

Smith, C.N., LaBrecque, G.C. & Borkovec, A.B. (1964) Insect chemosterilants. In: Smith, R.F. & Mittler, T.E., eds, Annual Review of Entomology, Palo Alto, California, Annual Reviews Inc., pp. 269-283

Terranova, A.C. (1969) Automated procedure for the determination of the aziridine moieties of N,N'-tetramethylenebis(1-aziridinecarboxamide) and other compounds containing aziridine. J. agric. Fd Chem., 17, 1047-1051

Truhaut, R., Delacoux, E., Brule, G. & Bohuon, C. (1963) Dosage des agents alcoylants dans les milieux biologiques. La méthode utilisant la réaction colorée avec la γ-(nitro-4-benzyl)-pyridine en milieu alcalin. Clin. chim. acta, 8, 235-245

2-METHYLAZIRIDINE

1. Chemical and Physical Data

1.1 Synonyms and trade names

Chem. Abstr. Reg. Serial No.:   75-55-8

Chem. Abstr. Name: 2-Methylaziridine

2-Methylazacyclopropane; methylethylenimine; propyleneimine;
1,2-propyleneimine; propylenimine; 1,2-propylenimine

1.2 Chemical formula and molecular weight

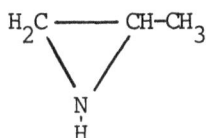

$$H_2C \text{------} CH\text{-}CH_3 \qquad\qquad C_3H_7N \qquad\qquad Mol.\ wt:\ 57.1$$

$$\diagdown\ \diagup$$

$$N$$
$$|$$
$$H$$

1.3 Chemical and physical properties of the pure substance

(a) Description: Colourless, oily liquid with odour like aliphatic
amines; fumes in air; flammable

(b) Boiling-point: 66-67°C at 760 mm Hg

(c) Melting-point: -65°C

(d) Density: d_4^{25} 0.802

(e) Refractive index: n_D^{25} 1.409

(f) Spectroscopy data: Extensive data have been compiled (Dermer &
Ham, 1969).

(g) Solubility: Miscible with water; soluble in ethanol

(h) Volatility: Vapour pressure is 112 mm Hg at 20°C.

(i) Stability: Polymerizes easily; hydrolyses in aqueous or
hydrochloric acid solutions to give methylethanolamine

(j) Reactivity: Reacts with carbonyl compounds, quinones and
sulphonyl halides

1.4 Technical products and impurities

High-purity 2-methylaziridine (inhibited with sodium hydroxide) is available in the US in 1-55 gallon drums, in 127 kg cylinders and in tank car or tank truck quantities (Anon., undated).

2. Production, Use, Occurrence and Analysis

For important background information on this section, see preamble p. 17.

2.1 Production and use

2-Methylaziridine can be prepared by the addition of hydrogen chloride to 1-amino-2-propanol to form 2-chloropropylamine hydrochloride, which is then treated with sodium hydroxide (Schaefer, 1955). It is manufactured commercially by combining 1,2-dichloropropane with ammonia at elevated temperatures (Dermer & Hart, 1966).

In 1965 there were two US manufacturers of this chemical (Dermer & Hart, 1966); however, at the present time, it is manufactured in commercial quantities by only one US manufacturer, and separate production data are not available. According to industry sources, 2-methylaziridine was produced commercially in Japan for several years in the 1960's.

2-Methylaziridine is apparently used in the US exclusively as an intermediate, since no evidence was found of its use in the monomeric form. Reactions with this chemical fall into two general groups: as a secondary amine yielding *N*-substituted propylene imines in which the ring is intact and as a cyclic amine involving ring opening reactions. Its main use is in the modification of latex surface coating resins to improve adhesion. Polymers modified with 2-methylaziridine or its derivatives have been used in the adhesive, textile and paper industries, because of the substantive bonding of imines to cellulose derivatives. 2-Methylaziridine has been used to modify dyes for specific adhesion to cellulose, and derivatives have also been used in photography, in gelatins and in synthetic resins. In the oil additive industry, this chemical and its derivatives have been used as modifiers for viscosity control, high pressure performance and oxidation resistance. Other uses have been in flocculants used in petroleum

62

refining, as a modifier for rocket propellant fuels, in fibre modification and in imine derivatives for use in human medicine and agricultural chemicals (Anon., undated). Its main use in Japan was probably in the treatment of paper.

2.2 Occurrence

2-Methylaziridine is not known to occur in nature.

The US Occupational Safety and Health Administration standards for occupational exposure to skin contaminants require that an employee's exposure to 2-methylaziridine not exceed 5 mg/m^3 (2 ppm) in air (US Code of Federal Regulations, 1973). A similar threshold limit value has been established in the Federal Republic of Germany (Anon., 1974).

2.3 Analysis

Gas chromatographic analysis (Di Lorenzo & Russo, 1968), thin-layer chromatography (Sawicki & Sawicki, 1969) and chromatographic separation of 2-methylaziridine on ion-exchange resins (Shimomura *et al.*, 1973) have been described.

3. Biological Data Relevant to the Evaluation of Carcinogenic Risk to Man

3.1 Carcinogenicity and related studies in animals

Oral administration

Rat: A group of 26 male and 26 female Charles River CD rats, 6 weeks of age, received 20 mg/kg bw 2-methylaziridine in water by gavage twice weekly for 28 weeks. Twenty-eight tumours were found within 60 weeks in 22/52 animals: 3 gliomas, 3 ear-duct squamous-cell carcinomas, 2 intestinal adenocarcinomas and 6 leukaemias occurred in males; and 10 breast tumours (mainly adenocarcinomas), 1 glioma and 3 miscellaneous tumours (not specified) occurred in females. In another group of 26 male and 26 female rats given 10 mg/kg bw for 60 weeks, 45 tumours were found in 37/52 animals: 4 gliomas, 3 ear-duct squamous-cell carcinomas, 2 intestinal adenocarcinomas, 4 leukaemias and 4 miscellaneous tumours (not specified) occurred in males; and 20 breast tumours, 2 gliomas, 3 ear-duct squamous-cell carcinomas and

3 miscellaneous tumours occurred in females. One pituitary adenoma was observed among 6 male and 6 female controls killed after 61 weeks (Ulland *et al.*, 1971).

3.2 Other relevant biological data

The toxicity of 2-methylaziridine is similar to that of aziridine. In rats, the oral LD_{50} has been reported to be 19 mg/kg bw; their exposure by inhalation to 500 ppm (1.2 mg/l) in air for 4 hours resulted in the death of most animals (Carpenter *et al.*, 1948).

3.3 Observations in man

No data were available to the Working Group.

4. Comments on Data Reported and Evaluation[1]

4.1 Animal data

2-Methylaziridine is carcinogenic in rats following its oral administration, the only species and route tested, producing a variety of malignant tumours.

4.2 Human data

No case reports or epidemiological studies were available to the Working Group.

---

[1]See also the section, "Animal Data in Relation to the Evaluation of Risk to Man" in the introduction to this volume, p. 15.

5. References

Anon. (undated) Organic Chemicals: Propylene Imine, Carlstadt, N.J., Arsynco Inc.

Anon. (1974) Maximale Arbeitsplatzkonzentrationen gesundheitschädlicher Stoffe, Koblenz, Bundesanstalt für Arbeitschutz und Unfallforschung

Carpenter, C.P., Smyth, H.F. & Shaffer, C.B. (1948) The acute toxicity of ethylene imine to small animals. J. industr. Hyg. Toxicol., 30, 2-6

Dermer, O.C. & Ham, G.L. (1969) Ethyleneimine and the Other Aziridines: Chemistry and Applications, New York, Academic Press

Dermer, O.C. & Hart, A.W. (1966) Imines, Cyclic. In: Kirk, R.E. & Othmer, D.F., eds, Encyclopedia of Chemical Technology, 2nd ed., Vol. 11, New York, John Wiley and Sons, pp. 526-548

Di Lorenzo, A. & Russo, G. (1968) Gas chromatographic analysis of aliphatic amines and imines. J. Gas Chromat., 6, 509-512

Sawicki, E. & Sawicki, C.R. (1969) Analysis of alkylating agents: applications to air pollution. Ann. N.Y. Acad. Sci., 163, 895-920

Schaefer, F.C. (1955) Homologs of triethylenemelamine. J. Amer. chem. Soc. 77, 5928-5929

Shimomura, K., Hsu, T.-J. & Walton, H.F. (1973) Ligand-exchange chromatography of aziridines and ethanolamines. Analyt. Chem., 45, 501-505

Ulland, B., Finkelstein, M., Weisburger, E.K., Rice, J.M. & Weisburger, J.H. (1971) Carcinogenicity of industrial chemicals propylene imine and propane sultone. Nature (Lond.), 230, 460-461

US Code of Federal Regulations (1973) Occupational Safety and Health Standards, Title 29, part 1910.93, Washington DC, US Government Printing Office, p. 21

TRIS(AZIRIDINYL)-*para*-BENZOQUINONE

1. Chemical and Physical Data

1.1 Synonyms and trade names

Chem. Abstr. Reg. Serial No.: 68-76-8

Chem. Abstr. Name: 2,3,5-Tris(1-aziridinyl)-2,5-cyclohexadiene-1,4-dione

1,1'1"-(3,6-Dioxo-1,4-cyclohexadiene-1,2,4-triyl)trisaziridine; TEIB; triaziquinone; triaziquone; triethyleneiminobenzoquinone; triethyleniminobenzoquinone; 2,3,5-triethylenimino-1,4-benzoquinone; 2,3,5-tris(aziridino)-1,4-benzoquinone; 2,3,5-tris(aziridinyl)-1,4-benzoquinone; 2,3,5-tris(1-aziridinyl)-*para*-benzoquinone; tris-(ethyleneimino)benzoquinone; 2,3,5-trisethyleneiminobenzoquinone; trisethyleneiminoquinone; 2,3,5-tris(ethylenimino)benzoquinone; 2,3,5-tris(ethylenimino)-1,4-benzoquinone; 2,3,5-tris(ethylenimino)-*para*-benzoquinone

Bayer 3231; Oncovedex; Prenimon; Riker 601; 10257 R.P.; Trenimon

1.2 Chemical formula and molecular weight

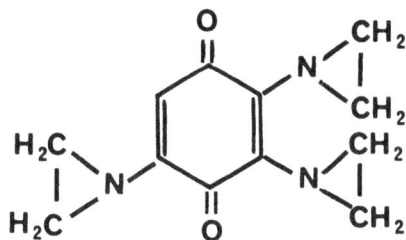

$C_{12}H_{13}N_3O_2$

Mol. wt: 231.2

1.3 Chemical and physical properties of the pure substance

(a) Description: Purple needles from ethyl acetate

(b) Melting-point: 162.5-163°C

(c) Solubility: Sparingly soluble in cold water; soluble in

acetone, benzene, chloroform, ethyl acetate, methanol and warm acetic acid

1.4 Technical products and impurities

Tris(1-aziridinyl)-*para*-benzoquinone (triaziquone) is available in dry form in ampoules containing 0.2 mg and as an oily suspension in enteric-coated capsules containing 0.5 mg (Blacow, 1967).

2. Production, Use, Occurrence and Analysis

For important background information on this section, see preamble, p. 17.

2.1 Production and use

Triaziquone can be prepared by the addition of 2,6-dimethoxy-1,4-benzoquinone to aziridine (Gauss & Domagk, 1961). No indication was found that it is produced in commercial quantities in the US, although it has been produced for research purposes. It is manufactured in the Federal Republic of Germany.

Triaziquone is used in the treatment of neoplastic diseases. The oral dosage varies from 0.5 mg/day to 1 mg/week; the i.v. dosage is usually 0.2 mg daily or every other day up to a total of 7 mg; and injections of 0.2-0.5 mg may be made into tumours. Triaziquone has been given intra-peritoneally at a dosage of 1-4 mg every 4 days, and also intrapleurally (Blacow, 1967).

This chemical has been tested in the US as an insect chemosterilant (Borkovec *et al.*, 1968), but it is believed that problems associated with its application to insects, its toxicity and environmental effects have prevented its use in this way on a commercial basis.

2.2 Occurrence

Triaziquone is not known to occur in nature.

2.3 Analysis

The colorimetric estimation of triaziquone in urine, blood and tissue extracts or homogenates using 4-(4'-nitrobenzyl)pyridine has been described

(Obrecht *et al.*, 1967); an automated colorimetric method using the same compound has also been described (Terranova, 1969).

3. Biological Data Relevant to the Evaluation of Carcinogenic Risk to Man

3.1 Carcinogenicity and related studies in animals

(a) Intravenous administration

Rat: Forty-eight male BR 46 rats, 100 days old, were injected intravenously once weekly with 0.03 mg/kg bw triaziquone (7% of the LD_{50}) for 52 weeks (total dose, 1.56 mg/kg bw). After 16±3 months, 11/45 (24%) animals had developed malignant tumours at various sites, and benign tumours were found in 4/45 animals. The malignant tumours were 5 sarcomas of the abdominal cavity, 1 lung squamous-cell carcinoma, 1 liver-cell carcinoma, 1 haemangiosarcoma of the salivary gland, 1 haemangiosarcoma of the kidney, 1 ear-duct carcinoma and 1 subcutaneous sarcoma. The benign tumours were 2 adenomas of the bronchus and 2 subcutaneous fibromas. After 23±5 months, 4/65 control rats had developed malignant tumours (3 mammary sarcomas and 1 phaeochromocytoma) and 3 animals had benign tumours (2 thymomas and 1 mammary fibroma) (Schmähl & Osswald, 1970). [P<0.02].

(b) Intravenous and intraperitoneal administration

Rat: Forty male BR 46 rats, 100 days of age, were injected intravenously once weekly with 0.03 mg/kg bw triaziquone for about 25 weeks. Thereafter the same dose was administered intraperitoneally for another 33 weeks (total dose, 1.74 mg/kg bw). After 16±2 months, 8 animals developed malignant tumours: 3 abdominal sarcomas, 1 reticulosarcomatosis, 1 myeloid leukaemia, 1 fibrosarcoma of the ribs, 1 lung carcinoma and 1 carcinoma of the kidney. Four animals had benign tumours: 1 an adenoma of the kidney in addition to a fibroma of the skin, 1 an adenoma of the bronchus, 1 a fibroma of the skin and 1 a thymoma. Among 50 control rats, 1 thymoma occurred within a period of 26 months (Schmähl, 1967).

3.2 Other relevant biological data

Klamerth & Kopun (1971) reported alkylation of DNA *in vitro* by triaziquone.

In *Saccharomyces cerevisiae*, triaziquone increased the gene conversion frequency by 100 times as compared to the spontaneous background at 32% inactivation (Zimmermann, 1971). In *Drosophila melanogaster* injected with triaziquone, the frequency of sex-chromosome loss and of the formation of sex-linked recessive lethals increased significantly (Mollet, 1973; Vogel, 1973). Chromosome aberrations in erythroblasts resulted in micronuclei in young polychromatic erythrocytes: in Chinese and Syrian golden hamsters, mice, rats and guinea-pigs a dose of 0.062 mg/kg bw resulted in a 5-10 times higher frequency of micronuclei than in controls. Similar results were obtained with 4 rhesus monkeys injected with 0.062 and 0.125 mg/kg bw (Matter & Schmid, 1971) and with ICR mice (von Ledebur & Schmid, 1973).

I.p. injection of triaziquone into male mice (Röhrborn, 1965) or female mice (Machemer & Hess, 1973; Röhrborn & Berrang, 1967) resulted in an increased frequency of dominant lethals. The doses ranged from 0.125-0.25 mg/kg bw; these were within the range of the clinical dose.

Human leucocytes treated with triaziquone *in vitro* showed a significant increase in the frequency of several different types of aberrations (Obe, 1968). The lowest effective dose for the induction of chromosome aberrations was 2.8×10^{-10} mol/l (Kaufmann *et al.*, 1973).

3.3 Observations in man

Three patients, one with an adenocarcinoma of the colon with metastases to the lung, one with a mammary carcinoma with metastases to the lymph nodes and one with a squamous-cell carcinoma of the bronchus without metastases, were treated with triaziquone for 52, 17 and 42 months, respectively. In one case androgens were given also. Leucopaenia was evident in all three cases, and at autopsy, 10 months to 4½ years after the end of treatment, atypical reticulum-cell growths described as "neoplastic reticulosis" were found in the bone marrow, spleen and lymph nodes (Terbrüggen, 1965). Treatment of a myosarcoma with triaziquone for 1½ years was associated with the later occurrence of a monocytic leukaemia; a course of radiation had been given also (Wildhack, 1970).

4. Comments on Data Reported and Evaluation[1]

4.1 Animal data

Tris(aziridinyl)-*para*-benzoquinone is carcinogenic in rats following its intravenous injection and also its intravenous followed by intraperitoneal administration, producing a variety of malignant tumours.

4.2 Human data

The four available case reports provide insufficient evidence on which to assess the carcinogenicity of this compound.

---

[1]See also the section, "Animal Data in Relation to the Evaluation of Risk to Man" in the introduction to this volume, p. 15.

5. References

Blacow, N.W., ed. (1967) Martindale: The Extra Pharmacopoeia, 25th ed., London, The Pharmaceutical Press

Borkovec, A.B., Fye, R.L. & LaBrecque, G.C. (1968) Aziridinyl chemosterilants for houseflies, ARS 33-129, Washington DC, US Department of Agriculture

Gauss, W. & Domagk, G. (1961) US Patent, 2,976,279, March 21, Schenley Industries Inc.

Kaufmann, W., Gebhart, E. & Horbach, L. (1973) Determination of the threshold value of the mutagenic activity of trenimon on human lymphocytes *in vitro*. Humangenetik, 20, 1-8

Klamerth, O.L. & Kopun, M. (1971) The influence of trenimon upon deoxyribonucleic acids *in vitro*. Europ. J. Biochem., 21, 199-203

von Ledebur, M. & Schmid, W. (1973) The micronucleus test. Methodological aspects. Mutation Res., 19, 109-117

Machemer, L. & Hess, R. (1973) Induced dominant lethals in female mice: effects of triaziquone and phenylbutazone. Experientia, 29, 190-192

Matter, B. & Schmid, W. (1971) Trenimon-induced chromosomal damage in bone-marrow cells of six mammalian species, evaluated by the micronucleus test. Mutation Res., 12, 417-425

Mollet, P. (1973) Untersuchungen über Mutagenität und Toxizität von Captan bei *Drosophila*. Mutation Res., 21, 132-148

Obe, G. (1968) Chemische Konstitution und mutagene Wirkung. V. Vergleichende Untersuchung der Wirkung von Äthyleniminen auf menschliche Leukozytenchromosomen. Mutation Res., 6, 467-471

Obrecht, P., Woenckhaus, J.W. & Fusenig, N.E. (1967) Die Verteilung von Trisaethyleniminobenzochinon (Trenimon) im Organismus der Ratte. Europ. J. Cancer, 3, 29-36

Röhrborn, G. (1965) Die mutagene Wirkung von Trenimon bei der männlichen Maus. Humangenetik, 1, 576-578

Röhrborn, G. & Berrang, H. (1967) Dominant lethals in young female mice. Mutation Res., 4, 231-233

Schmähl, D. (1967) Karzinogene Wirkung von Cyclophosphamid und Triazichon bei Ratten. Dtsch. med. Wschr., 92, 1150-1152

Schmähl, D. & Osswald, H. (1970) Experimentelle Untersuchungen über carcinogene Wirkungen von Krebs-Chemotherapeutica und Immunosuppressiva. Arzneimittel-Forsch., 20, 1461-1467

Terbrüggen, A. (1965) Neoplastische Retikulose nach zytostatischer Dauer-
    behandlung von radikal operierten Karzinomen. Dtsch. Ges. Path., 49,
    241-245

Terranova, A.C. (1969) Automated procedure for the determination of the
    aziridine moieties of N,N'-tetramethylenebis(1-aziridinecarboxamide)
    and other compounds containing aziridine. J. agric. Fd Chem., 17,
    1047-1051

Vogel, E. (1973) Strong antimutagenic effects of fluoride on mutation
    induction by trenimon and 1-phenyl-3,3-dimethyltriazene in *Drosophila
    melanogaster*. Mutation Res., 20, 339-352

Wildhack, R. (1970) Monozytenleukämie mit γG-Paraproteinämie nach Röntgen-
    nachbestrahlung und zytostatischer Behandlung eines Myosarkoms.
    Dtsch. med. Wschr., 92, 255-257

Zimmermann, F.K. (1971) Induction of mitotic gene conversion by mutagens.
    Mutation Res., 11, 327-337

TRIS(1-AZIRIDINYL)PHOSPHINE OXIDE

1. Chemical and Physical Data

1.1 Synonyms and trade names

Chem. Abstr. Reg. Serial No.:   545-55-1

Chem. Abstr. Name: 1,1',1"-Phosphinylidynetrisaziridine

Aphoxide; APO; ENT-24915; phosphoric acid triethylene imide; TEF; TEPA; tepa; triaziridinylphosphine oxide; N,N',N''-tri-1,2-ethane-diylphosphoric triamide; triethylenephosphamide; N,N',N''-triethylene-phosphoramide; triethylenephosphoric triamide; N,N',N''-triethylene-phosphoric triamide; triethylenephosphorotriamide; triethylenepyro-phosphoramide; tris(aziridinyl)phosphine oxide

SK-3818

1.2 Chemical formula and molecular weight

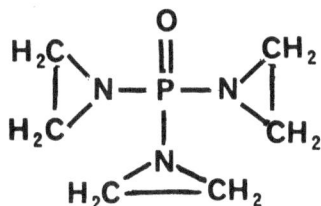

$C_6H_{12}N_3OP$

Mol. wt: 173.2

1.3 Chemical and physical properties of the pure substance

(a) Description: Colourless crystals; very hygroscopic

(b) Melting-point: $41^{\circ}C$

(c) Boiling-point: $90-91^{\circ}C$ at 23 mm Hg

(d) Spectroscopy data: The infrared spectrum has been reported (Spell, 1967).

(e) Solubility: Very soluble in water, ethanol, ether and acetone

(f) Stability: Stable in aqueous solution at low temperature, but rapidly degraded by boiling. At an initial pH of 6.8 and temperatures of 3, 25, 50 and 100°C, the half-lives of 0.3% solutions of tris(1-aziridinyl)phosphine oxide (tepa) in terms of imine function were >200, 31, 7 and <0.1 days, respectively. The rate of degradation of tepa was pH-dependent: it was relatively stable at pH 9 but degraded rapidly at pH 4 (Beroza & Borkovec, 1964).

For long-term storage, tepa has been suspended in sesame oil under unspecified conditions; however, some degradation was noted after 22 months (Thiersch, 1957). Storage has been achieved using anhydrous polyethyleneglycol (Nakabayashi, 1960).

(g) Reactivity: Decomposes in acid solution with the formation of aziridine; NMR spectroscopy revealed other decomposition products which were attributed to the opening of aziridine rings rather than to cleavage of P-N bonds. During slower degradation in alkaline solution, aziridine itself was not observed (Beroza & Borkovec, 1964). Ring opening has also been observed on reaction with carboxylic acids (Brock, 1963, quoted in Dermer & Ham, 1969).

1.4 Technical products and impurities

No data were available to the Working Group.

2. Production, Use, Occurrence and Analysis

For important background information on this section, see preamble, p. 17.

2.1 Production and use

Tepa can be prepared by the addition of aziridine to phosphorous oxychloride (Bestian, 1950). It has been estimated that approximately 400,000 kg of the chemical were consumed in the US in the late 1960's for flame-retardant treatment of military cotton. Its use in this application was terminated when the sole US commercial manufacturer discontinued production for economic reasons (Lyons, 1970).

Industry sources report that several hundred kg per month of tepa were manufactured by one company in Japan in the late 1960's and early 1970's, all of which was apparently exported to the US for use in textile applications. Tepa is produced in the Federal Republic of Germany (Chemical Information Services, Ltd, 1975).

Clinical trials of tepa as an antineoplastic agent were reported in the US in 1953 (Farber *et al.*, 1953). Although it was tested in animals and humans, it was never extensively used in cancer therapy due to the discovery of an equally effective but less toxic sulphur analogue, tris-(1-aziridinyl)phosphine sulphide (Smith *et al.*, 1964).

Although tepa was shown to be effective as a chemosterilant for a variety of insects (Smith *et al.*, 1964), problems associated with its application to insects, its toxicity and environmental effects have prevented its use in this way on a commercial basis.

Tepa has been used as an acaricide, in the permanent press treatment of cotton (Lyons, 1970), in textile dyeing, in polymer stabilization, as a photographic emulsion hardener (Stecher, 1968) and as a modifier to increase specific adhesion to certain substrates (Dermer & Hart, 1966). It has also been used to impart permanent flame resistance to cotton fabrics by reaction with tetrakis(hydroxymethyl)phosphonium chloride (Drake *et al.*, 1961).

2.2 Occurrence

Tepa is not known to occur in nature.

2.3 Analysis

A titration procedure based on the reaction of the aziridine groups with thiosulphate has been used for the determination of tepa in solution (Allen & Seaman, 1955). Colour reactions using 4-(4'-nitrobenzyl)pyridine have also been used (Epstein *et al.*, 1955; Preussmann *et al.*, 1969; Terranova, 1969). The separation of tepa from preparations of pulverized insects prior to its determination by colorimetric procedures has been achieved by the use of columns containing anhydrous sodium sulphate and silica gel (Collier & Tardif, 1967).

Solvent systems suitable for use in the identification of urinary metabolites by paper chromatography have been reported (Craig & Jackson,

1955; Nadkarni *et al.*, 1957). Thin-layer systems on plates of silica gel have been developed; those spots containing aziridine functions have been identified using 4-(4'-nitrobenzyl)pyridine (Beroza & Borkovec, 1964) and 4-pyridinealdehyde-2-benzothiazolylhydrazone and 4-pyridinealdehyde-4-nitrophenylhydrazone, sensitive to 0.2 and 1 μg, respectively (Sawicki & Sawicki, 1969).

A spectrophotofluorimetric method, suitable for determinations in 0.05-0.2 μg/ml body fluid, has been used to determine tepa in the presence of tris(1-aziridinyl)phosphine sulphide in extracts of biological tissues and fluids. Separation is based upon the differential solubility of these two phosphoramides in benzene during the extraction of aqueous samples (Mellett & Woods, 1960).

NMR spectroscopy has proved useful in studies of the degradation products of tepa. The intact compound has a characteristic doublet signal, and singlets are not observed until P-N bonds have been broken (Beroza & Borkovec, 1964).

More recently, gas chromatographic procedures have provided methods of analysis sensitive to 0.1 ng. Retention times for tepa have been reported (Bowman & Beroza, 1970), and a procedure directly applicable to methanolic extracts of insect tissues has been described (Seawright *et al.*, 1971). A useful micro-test (not specific for tepa), sensitive to 1 μg, can be made by reaction with thiosulphate in the presence of a mixed indicator solution, followed by the addition of sulphuric acid (Beroza & Borkovec, 1964).

3. Biological Data Relevant to the Evaluation of Carcinogenic Risk to Man

3.1 Carcinogenicity and related studies in animals

Oral administration

Rat: Six groups of weanling male and female Fischer rats were given daily doses of 0.001-0.3 mg tepa in steroid suspending vehicle* by gavage

---

*NaCl, Na carboxymethylcellulose, Polysorbate 80, benzyl alcohol and water

on 5 days per week for 1 year. The average survival times were 240 and 500 days for the two highest dose groups and 560 days for the other treated groups. Of 58 treated animals, 34 developed tumours: 1 adenocarcinoma, 1 fibrosarcoma and 6 fibroadenomas of the mammary gland, 10 interstitial-cell tumours and 1 mesothelioma of the testis, 1 fibroma and 1 fibrosarcoma, 1 lung adenoma, 1 hepatoma, 2 bronchial adenomas, 2 squamous-cell carcinomas of the ear, 1 skin papilloma, 3 lymphomas, 2 others and 1 basal-cell carcinoma of the lip, which was the only tumour observed at the area of application. In 653 controls, only 56 tumours were observed at sites other than the testis; the incidence of interstitial-cell tumours of the testis was 25/26 in males examined at 600 days; mammary fibroadenomas were infrequent, being found mostly in old females (5/160 in rats killed between 531 and 600 days) (Hadidian *et al.*, 1968).

3.2 Other relevant biological data

In rats, the LD_{50} by oral administration is 37 mg/kg bw (Stecher, 1968) and by skin application, 87 mg/kg bw. In the rabbit, the maximum tolerated single dose was 5 mg/kg bw when given intramuscularly and 0.5 mg/kg bw orally (Schmidt, 1954).

After i.p. administration of ^{32}P-tepa to mice, radioactivity was not localized selectively in any of the tissues examined. During the first 24 hours after treatment some 60-75% of the dose was excreted *via* the urine, compared with only 2-5% in faeces. In urine, 80% of the radioactivity was identified as inorganic phosphate, the remainder as an unidentified metabolite which could be hydrolysed to give organic phosphate (Nadkarni *et al.*, 1957).

In rats, 80% of the radioactivity in blood was associated with haemoglobin. During the first 24 hours 89-90% of the radioactivity was excreted in the urine; however, in contrast with the mouse, 50-70% of the urinary radioactivity was present as unchanged tepa (Craig & Jackson, 1955).

The pattern of metabolism in dogs is essentially similar to that described for rats. Recovery of unchanged tepa in urine was about 25-30% of the dose over the same period. Tissue distribution studies showed that retention was uniformly low, with the exception of bone marrow in which selective uptake resulted in a concentration six to ten times that found in other tissues (Mellett & Woods, 1960).

Sherman rats were treated i.p. with 5-10 mg/kg bw on the 11th day of pregnancy: the higher doses were toxic to the mothers and caused some foetal resorptions and decreased foetal and placental weight. At doses tolerated by the mothers many resorptions were observed; but, in contrast with the effects of tris(2-methyl-1-aziridinyl)phosphine oxide, no malformations were seen (Kimbrough & Gaines, 1968). Freshly-prepared suspensions of 5 mg/kg bw tepa in sesame oil given intramuscularly to Wistar rats on the 4th and 5th, 7th and 8th or 11th and 12th days of gestation caused resorption of almost all foetuses (Thiersch, 1957).

Tepa induces back-mutations of an auxotrophic strain of *Schizosaccharomyces pombe* (Zetterberg, 1971), dominant lethals in *Musca domestica* (LaChance & Leopold, 1969) and dominant lethals, sex-linked recessive lethals and Y-II-III chromosome translocations in *Drosophila melanogaster* (Srám, 1972).

Frequencies of dominant lethals were significantly increased in the progeny of male Swiss mice given i.p. injections of tepa at doses ranging from 0.156-20 mg/kg bw (Epstein *et al.*, 1970). Srám *et al.* (1970a) obtained similar results in A/L and C57BL/6J mice. CD rats given an i.p. injection of 10 mg/kg bw tepa had chromatid aberrations in 87.5% of bone-marrow cells (Adler *et al.*, 1971).

Induction of transmissible translocations has been found after single i.p. injections of tepa in male Swiss albino (Epstein *et al.*, 1971) and A/L mice (Srám *et al.*, 1970b). A high frequency of chromosome aberrations was observed *in vitro* after treatment of human leucocyte cultures with tepa (Chang & Klassen, 1968).

The metabolism of tepa in man is similar to that described for mice (Nadkarni *et al.*, 1959).

3.3 Observations in man

No data were available to the Working Group.

4. Comments on Data Reported and Evaluation

4.1 Animal data

Tris(1-aziridinyl)phosphine oxide produced a low incidence of benign and malignant tumours in rats following its oral administration, the only species and route tested. The available data are insufficient for evaluation of the carcinogenicity of this compound.

4.2 Human data

No case reports or epidemiological studies were available to the Working Group.

5. References

Adler, I.D., Ramarao, G. & Epstein, S.S. (1971) *In vivo* cytogenetic effects of trimethylphosphate and of TEPA on bone marrow cells of male rats. Mutation Res., 13, 263-273

Allen, E. & Seaman, W. (1955) Method of assay for ethylenimine derivatives. Analyt. Chem., 27, 540-543

Beroza, M. & Borkovec, A.B. (1964) The stability of tepa and other aziridine chemosterilants. J. med. Chem., 7, 44-49

Bestian, H. (1950) Über einige Reaktionen des Äthylen-imine. Ann. Chem., 566, 210-215

Bowman, M.C. & Beroza, M. (1970) GLC retention times of pesticides and metabolites containing phosphorus and sulphur on four thermally stable columns. J. Ass. off. analyt. Chem., 53, 499-508

Chang, T.-H. & Klassen, W. (1968) Comparative effects of tretamine, TEPA, apholate and their structural analogs on human chromosomes *in vitro*. Chromosoma (Berl.), 24, 314-323

Chemical Information Services, Ltd (1975) Directory of Western European Chemical Producers, 1975/76, Oceanside, N.Y.

Collier, C.W. & Tardif, R. (1967) Analysis of male gypsy moths for microgram quantities of tepa. J. econ. Entomol., 60, 28-30

Craig, A.W. & Jackson, H. (1955) The metabolism of ^{32}P-labelled triethylenephosphoramide in relation to its anti-tumour activity. Brit. J. Pharmacol., 10, 321-325

Dermer, O.C. & Ham, G.E. (1969) Ethyleneimine and Other Aziridines: Chemistry and Applications, New York, Academic Press, p. 259

Dermer, O.C. & Hart, A.W. (1966) Imines, Cyclic. In: Kirk, R.E. & Othmer, D.F., eds, Encyclopedia of Chemical Technology, 2nd ed., Vol. 11, New York, John Wiley and Sons, pp. 526-548

Drake, G.L., Jr, Beninate, J.V. & Guthrie, J.D. (1961) Application of the APO-THPC flame retardant to cotton fabric. American Dyestuff Reporter, 50, 129-134

Epstein, J., Rosenthal, R.W. & Ess, R.J. (1955) Use of γ-(4-nitrobenzyl)-pyridine as analytical reagent for ethylenimines and alkylating agents. Analyt. Chem., 27, 1435-1439

Epstein, S.S., Arnold, E., Steinberg, K., Mackintosh, D., Shafner, H. & Bishop, Y. (1970) Mutagenic and antifertility effects of TEPA and METEPA in mice. Toxicol. appl. Pharmacol., 17, 23-40

Epstein, S.S., Bass, W., Arnold, E., Bishop, Y., Joshi, S. & Adler, I.D. (1971) Sterility and semisterility in male progeny of male mice treated with the chemical mutagen TEPA. Toxicol. appl. Pharmacol., 19, 134-146

Farber, S., Appleton, R., Downing, V., Heald, F., King, J. & Toch, R. (1953) Clinical studies on the carcinolytic action of triethylenephosphoramide. Cancer, 6, 135-141

Hadidian, Z., Fredrickson, T.N., Weisburger, E.K., Weisburger, J.H., Glass, R.M. & Mantel, N. (1968) Tests for chemical carcinogens. Report on the activity of derivatives of aromatic amines, nitrosamines, quinolines, nitroalkanes, amides, epoxides, aziridines and purine antimetabolites. J. nat. Cancer Inst., 41, 985-1036

Kimbrough, R.D. & Gaines, T.B. (1968) Effect of organic phosphorus compounds and alkylating agents on the rat fetus. Arch. environm. Hlth, 16, 805-808

LaChance, L.E. & Leopold, R.A. (1969) Cytogenetic effects of chemosterilants in house fly sperm: incidence of polyspermy and expression of dominant lethal mutations in early cleavage divisions. Canad. J. Genet. Cytol., 11, 648-659

Lyons, J.W. (1970) The Chemistry and Uses of Fire Retardants, New York, Interscience, pp. 174-179

Mellett, L.B. & Woods, L.A. (1960) The comparative physiological disposition of thioTEPA and TEPA in the dog. Cancer Res., 20, 524-532

Nadkarni, M.V., Goldenthal, E.I. & Smith, P.K. (1957) The distribution of radioactivity following administration of triethylenephosphoramide-P^{32} in tumor-bearing and control mice. Cancer Res., 17, 97-101

Nadkarni, M.V., Trams, E.G. & Smith, P.K. (1959) Preliminary studies on the distribution and fate of TEM, TEPA and myleran in the human. Cancer Res., 19, 713-718

Nakabayashi, K. (1960) Stable injection solution from tablets containing ethyleneimine derivatives. Japanese Patent, 13,943, September 22, Sumito Chemical Industry Co., Ltd

Preussmann, R., Schneider, H. & Epple, F. (1969) Untersuchungen zum Nachweis alkylierender Agentien. II. Der Nachweis verschiedener Klassen alkylierender Agentien mit einer Modifikation der Farbreaktion mit 4-(4-Nitrobenzyl)-pyridin. Arzneimittel-Forsch., 19, 1059-1073

Sawicki, E. & Sawicki, C.R. (1969) Analysis of alkylating agents: applications to air pollution. Ann. N.Y. Acad. Sci., 163, 895-920

Schmidt, K.H. (1954) Experimentelle und vergleichende Ergebnisse mit Triäthylenmelamin, *N,N',N"*-Triäthylenphosphorsäureamid und 6-Mercaptopurin. Arzneimittel-Forsch., 4, 146-161

Seawright, J.A., Bowman, M.C. & Patterson, R.S. (1971) Tepa and thiotepa: uptake, persistence and stability induced in pupae and adults of *Culex pipiens quinquefasciatus*. J. econ. Entomol., 64, 452-455

Smith, C.N., LaBrecque, G.C. & Borkovec, A.B. (1964) Insect chemosterilants. In: Smith, R.F. & Mittler, T.E., eds, Annual Review of Entomology, Vol. 9, Palo Alto, California, Annual Reviews Inc., pp. 269-284

Spell, H.L. (1967) The infra-red spectra of *N*-substituted aziridine compounds. Analyt. Chem., 39, 185-193

Srám, R.J. (1972) The differences in the spectra of genetic changes in *Drosophila melanogaster* induced by chemosterilants TEPA and HEMPA. Folia biol. (Praha), 18, 139-148

Srám, R.J., Benes, V. & Zudova, Z. (1970a) Induction of dominant lethals in mice by TEPA and HEMPA. Folia biol. (Praha), 16, 407-416

Srám, R.J., Zudova, Z. & Benes, V. (1970b) Induction of translocations in mice by TEPA. Folia biol. (Praha), 16, 367-368

Stecher, P.G., ed. (1968) The Merck Index, 8th ed., Rahway, N.J., Merck & Co., p. 1073

Terranova, A.C. (1969) Automated procedure for the determination of the aziridine moieties of *N,N'*-tetramethylenebis(1-aziridinecarboxamide) and other compounds containing aziridine. J. agric. Fd Chem., 17, 1047-1051

Thiersch, J.B. (1957) Effect of 2,4,6-triamino-S-triazine (TR), 2,4,6-tris(ethylenimino)-S-triazine (TEM) and *N,N',N"*-triethylenephosphoramide (TEPA) on rat litter *in utero*. Proc. Soc. exp. Biol. (N.Y.), 94, 36-40

Zetterberg, G. (1971) Bacteriophage development in lysogenic *Escherichia coli* and mutations in fungi induced with analogs of tris(1-aziridinyl)-phosphine oxide, TEPA. Hereditas, 68, 245-254

84

TRIS (1-AZIRIDINYL)PHOSPHINE SULPHIDE

1. Chemical and Physical Data

1.1 Synonyms and trade names

Chem. Abstr. Reg. Serial No.: 52-24-4

Chem. Abstr. Name: 1,1',1"-Phosphinothioylidynetrisaziridine

Thiophosphamide; thiotepa; thiotriethylenephosphoramide; tri-aziridinylphosphine sulphide; $N,N',N"$-tri-1,2-ethanediylphosphoro-thioic triamide; $N,N',N"$-tri-1,2-ethanediylthiophosphoramide; tri-(ethyleneimino)thiophosphoramide; $N,N',N"$-triethylenephosphorothioic triamide; triethylenethiophosphoramide; $N,N',N"$-triethylenethio-phosphoramide; triethylenethiophosphorotriamide; tris(ethylenimino)-thiophosphate

Girostan; Oncotepa; TESPA; Tespamine; Thio-TEP; Thio-TEPA; Tifosyl; TSPA

1.2 Chemical formula and molecular weight

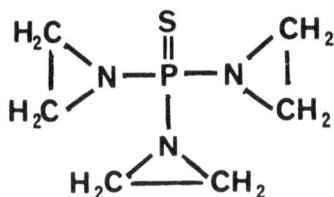

$C_6H_{12}N_3PS$

Mol. wt: 189.2

1.3 Chemical and physical properties of the pure substance

(a) Description: White, crystalline solid

(b) Melting-point: 51.5°C

(c) Solubility: 19 g/100 ml water at 25°C; freely soluble in ethanol; soluble in ether, benzene and chloroform

(d) Stability: Dilute aqueous solutions (0.1%) are stable for months at temperatures below 20°C; for 45 hours at 30°C; for 2 hours in the presence of oxygen, carbon dioxide or light; and for 30 minutes when exposed to UV-light; boiling for 10 minutes inactivates 35% of the agent (Lidaks *et al.*, 1959). Unstable at pH 4.2; its destruction is therefore to be expected in the human stomach (Mellett & Woods, 1960). In dilute solution at pH 1 hydrogen sulphide is released ($t_{\frac{1}{2}}$, approx. 3 hours) (Benckhuijsen, 1968).

1.4 Technical products and impurities

Tris (l-aziridinyl)phosphine sulphide (thiotepa) is available in 15 mg vials containing 97-102% active ingredient. It can also be obtained as a sterile mixture for injection containing 1 part thiotepa, 5.3 parts sodium chloride and 3.3 parts sodium bicarbonate; in this form, the product contains 95-110% of the labelled amount of active ingredient (15 mg) and is available as a powder in ampoules (US Pharmacopeial Convention, Inc., 1970).

2. Production, Use, Occurrence and Analysis

For important background information on this section, see preamble, p. 17.

2.1 Production and use

Thiotepa can be prepared by the addition of trichlorophosphine sulphide to aziridine and triethylamine (Kuh & Seeger, 1954). There is only one producer of thiotepa in the United States, and so production data are not reported. Industry sources report that one Japanese manufacturer formerly produced small quantities for trial purposes. This chemical is marketed as an antineoplastic drug in Belgium and Sweden (Société Suisse de Pharmacie, 1973).

The only known commercial use for thiotepa in the US is as an antineoplastic agent, and investigation of its use in the treatment of leukaemia is believed to have been the first trial in cancer therapy research (Shay *et al.*, 1953). In 1957 it was listed as a commonly used alkylating agent for cancer therapy (Endicott, 1957), but by 1973 only 3 kg were used for antineoplastic purposes in the US. The most consistent results with this drug have been obtained in the treatment of the following tumours: adenocarcinoma of the breast, adenocarcinoma of the ovary, malignant lymphomas (giant follicular lymphoma, lymphosarcoma, reticulum-cell sarcoma, Hodgkin's disease), bronchogenic carcinoma and Wilm's tumour (Medical Economics Co., 1974; Wright *et al.*, 1958). Recommended initial dosage in adults is 60 mg, with maintenance dosage adjusted to patient requirements (Medical Economics Co., 1974). Thiotepa has also been used in combination with melphalan (Krementz & Ryan, 1972).

Thiotepa was tested extensively for use as an intermediate in the manufacture of polymeric flame retardants for cotton (Reeves *et al.*, 1957); but it has probably not been used commercially in this way in either the US or the UK.

Thiotepa has been shown to be an effective insect chemosterilant (Knipling *et al.*, 1968; Patterson *et al.*, 1971; Smith *et al.*, 1964; White, 1966), but problems associated with its application to insects, its toxicity and environmental effects have prevented its use in this way on a commercial basis.

2.2 Occurrence

Thiotepa is not known to occur in nature.

2.3 Analysis

A variety of procedures are available for the determination of thiotepa in extracts of body fluids and tissues. Colorimetric determinations using 4-(4'-nitrobenzyl)pyridine have been described (Butler *et al.*, 1967; Epstein *et al.*, 1955; Klatt *et al.*, 1960; Tan & Cole, 1965; Truhaut *et al.*, 1963), and the use of Dragendorff and Nessler reagents has been reported (Buchkova *et al.*, 1972). Other methods of analysis include a sensitive spectrophotofluorimetric procedure (range, 0.05-0.2 µg/ml body fluid) (Mellett & Woods, 1960); paper chromatography (Bateman *et al.*, 1960; Craig *et al.*, 1959); thin-layer chromatography (Benckhuijsen, 1968; Mirkina & Kharlamov, 1965); titration employing thiosulphate (Allen & Seaman, 1955; Raine, 1962) or thiocyanate (Ozolins & Egerts, 1968); and electrochemical procedures (Inkin *et al.*, 1968; Nangniot, 1966). The most sensitive methods are gas chromatographic techniques, capable of detecting sub-ng quantities, which were developed in order to follow the absorption and retention of thiotepa in insects during studies related to

the use of the drug as a chemosterilant (Bowman & Beroza, 1970; Seawright
et al., 1971). Ion-exchange chromatography procedures, which may be poten-
tially useful in the identification of metabolites, have also been described
(Plapp & Casida, 1958). Thiotepa may also be assayed by proton magnetic
resonance (Cates, 1973).

3. Biological Data Relevant to the Evaluation
of Carcinogenic Risk to Man

3.1 Carcinogenicity and related studies in animals

(a) Intraperitoneal administration

Mouse: Three groups of 20 male and female A/He mice, 6-8 weeks old,
were treated with thiotepa in tricaprylin intraperitoneally thrice weekly
for a total of 12 injections. After 24 weeks, total doses of 19, 47 and
94 mg/kg bw had produced 0.70, 0.74 and 1.50 lung adenomas per mouse in
11/20, 20/20 and 16/20 mice, respectively. In controls, 28% and 20% of
77 males and 77 females had developed lung tumours with frequencies of
0.24 and 0.20 lung tumours per mouse. In these tests thiotepa was 20 times
less active on a molar basis than uracil mustard (Stoner *et al.*, 1973).

(b) Intravenous administration

Rat: Thiotepa was administered to 100-day old BR 46 rats at 7% of
the LD_{50} (1 mg/kg bw) once weekly for 52 weeks. Malignant tumours developed
in 9/30 (30%) treated animals: 2 sarcomas of the abdominal cavity, 1
lymphosarcoma, 1 seminoma, 1 haemangioendothelioma, 1 fibrosarcoma of the
salivary gland, 1 sarcoma of the mammary gland, 1 pheochromocytoma and
1 myelosis; 5/30 (17%) had benign tumours. In controls, malignant tumours
were found in 4/65 (6%) animals: 3 sarcomas of the mammary gland and 1
pheochromocytoma; and benign tumours were seen in 3/65 (5%) animals
(Schmähl & Osswald, 1970) [P<0.01].

3.2 Other relevant biological data

The LD_{50} in rats was about 9 mg/kg bw when given either by the i.v.
or i.a. route (Boone *et al.*, 1962). The oral LD_{50} in mice is 46 mg/kg bw
(Stecher, 1968). Pentobarbital given concomittantly reduced the LD_{50} of
thiotepa in mice (Munson *et al.*, 1974).

In mice, thiotepa is rapidly metabolized to tris (1-aziridinyl)phosphine oxide (tepa): within 30 minutes only tepa and inorganic phosphate were detected in the urine and plasma. The mouse is exceptional in its ability to degrade the drug completely to inorganic phosphate (Craig et al., 1959).

In rats, thiotepa was evenly distributed throughout the organs, but the highest proportion was found in the liver(Craig et al., 1959). Most of the drug and its principal metabolite, tepa, are excreted in the urine during the first few hours (Boone et al., 1962), but a small fraction of radioactivity was retained in blood haemoglobin after 9 days.

In rabbits and dogs the main urinary metabolite was tepa, and only trace amounts of inorganic phosphate were found in the urine (Craig et al., 1959; Mellett et al., 1962).

Thiotepa was teratogenic in pregnant mice injected intraperitoneally with single doses of 0.5-30 mg/kg bw on various days of gestation. The minimum teratogenic dose was 1 mg/kg bw; after administration of 10 mg/kg bw all foetuses were malformed (Tanimura, 1968). After rats were given 5 mg/kg bw thiotepa, gross developmental abnormalities and skeletal defects were observed in foetuses (Murphy et al., 1958).

Thiotepa increased the frequency of inherited recessive lethals in *Drosophila melanogaster* (Lüers & Röhrborn, 1965). Treatment of male CFLP mice with single i.p. injections of 5 or 10 mg/kg bw thiotepa induced a high frequency of dominant lethals (Machemer & Hess, 1971). Insemination of female rabbits with sperm treated with thiotepa *in vitro* led to a high increase in the frequency of dominant lethals (Nuzhdin & Nizhnik, 1968). Treatment with this chemical of cultured human lymphocytes resulted in a significant increase in the frequency of chromosome aberrations (Bochkov & Kuleshov, 1972; Hampel et al., 1966).

In man, 50% of an injection of ^{14}C-thiotepa either intravenously or locally into the tumour was excreted in the first 6 hours, and by 48 hours only low levels persisted (Bateman et al., 1960). Absorption of an orally administered dose of ^{14}C-thiotepa was variable: less than 1% of the injected dose was recovered as unchanged drug in the urine (Mellett et al., 1962).

The major metabolite of thiotepa, tepa, has also been tested for carcinogenicity in experimental animals (see p. 75).

3.3 Observations in man

At least 9 cases of acute leukaemia (7 myeloblastic, 1 myelomonocytic, 1 erythromegakaryocytic) have been reported in patients with malignancies of the ovary, breast or lung who had been treated with thiotepa for 13-60 months (Allan, 1970; Garfield, 1970; Greenspan & Tung, 1974; Kaslow *et al.*, 1972; Perlman & Walker, 1973; Ruffner, 1974; Solomon & Firat, 1971; Sypkens-Smit & Meyler, 1970). In 6 of the cases, thiotepa was used with other chemotherapeutic agents and/or radiation. The interval between first administration of the drug and diagnosis of leukaemia was 30-84 months. The occurrence of two cases of acute leukaemia among 400 patients with ovarian cancer described by Greenspan & Tung (1974) suggests an increased incidence of acute leukaemia among women with ovarian cancer given chemo-therapeutic regimens which include thiotepa.

4. Comments on Data Reported and Evaluation[1]

4.1 Animal data

Tris(1-aziridinyl)phosphine sulphide is carcinogenic in mice following its intraperitoneal injection and in rats following its intravenous injection, producing a dose-related increase in the incidence of lung tumours in mice and a variety of malignant tumours in rats.

4.2 Human data

Reports of 9 cases of acute leukaemia following previous therapuetic use of thiotepa suggest an association, but they provide insufficient evidence on which to assess the carcinogenic risk of this compound.

---

[1]See also the section, "Animal Data in Relation to the Evaluation of Risk to Man" in the introduction to this volume, p. 15.

5. References

Allan, W.S.A. (1970) Acute myeloid leukaemia after treatment with cyto-
    static agents. Lancet, ii, 775

Allen, E. & Seaman, W. (1955) Method of assay for ethylenimine derivatives.
    Analyt. Chem., 27, 540-543

Bateman, J.C., Carlton, H.N., Calvert, R.C. & Lindenblad, G.E. (1960)
    Investigation of distribution and excretion of ^{14}C-tagged triethylene
    thiophosphoramide following injection by various routes. Int. J. appl.
    Radiat., 7, 287-298

Benckhuijsen, C. (1968) Acid-catalysed conversion of triethyleneimine
    thiophosphoramide (thio-TEPA) to an SH compound. Biochem. Pharmacol.,
    17, 55-64

Bochkov, N.P. & Kuleshov, N.P. (1972) Age sensitivity of human chromosomes
    to alkylating agents. Mutation Res., 14, 345-353

Boone, I.U., Rogers, B.S. & Williams, D.L. (1962) Toxicity, metabolism and
    tissue distribution of carbon^{14}-labelled N,N',N''-triethylenethiophos-
    phoramide (thio-TEPA) in rats. Toxicol. appl. Pharmacol., 4, 344-353

Bowman, M.C. & Beroza, M. (1970) GLC retention times of pesticides and
    metabolites containing phosphorus and sulfur on four thermally stable
    columns. J. Ass. off. analyt. Chem., 53, 499-508

Buchkova, M.N., Koval'chuk, T.V. & Shakh, T.I. (1972) Methods of examina-
    tion of ethylenimine derivative drugs. Farm. Zh. (Kiev), 27, 24-30

Butler, C.G., Kaushik, D.S., Maxwell, J. & Stell, J.G.P. (1967) The
    colorimetric estimation of thiotepa. J. mond. Pharm., 10, 350-364

Cates, L.A. (1973) Assay of thiotepa by PMR spectrometry. J. Pharm. Sci.,
    62, 1698-1699

Craig, A.W., Fox, B.W. & Jackson, H. (1959) Metabolic studies of ^{32}P-
    labeled triethylenethiophosphoramide. Biochem. Pharmacol., 3, 42-50

Endicott, K.M. (1957) Current chemotherapy for cancer. Modern Med.,
    November 15, pp. 260, 263, 266, 269

Epstein, J., Rosenthal, R.W. & Ess, R.J. (1955) Use of γ-(4-nitrobenzyl)-
    pyridine as analytical reagent for ethylenimines and alkylating agents.
    Analyt. Chem., 27, 1435-1439

Garfield, D.H. (1970) Acute erythromegakaryocytic leukaemia after treat-
    ment with cytostatic agents. Lancet, ii, 1037

Greenspan, E.M. & Tung, B.G. (1974) Acute myeloblastic leukaemia after cure of ovarian cancer. J. Amer. med. Ass., 230, 418-420

Hampel, K.E., Kober, B., Rösch, D., Gerhartz, H. & Meinig, K.-H. (1966) The action of cytostatic agents on the chromosomes of human leukocytes *in vitro* (preliminary communication). Blood, 27, 816-823

Inkin, A.A., Kharlamov, V.T. & Tsimbalaev, R.M. (1968) Coulometric titration of thio-TEPA [tris(1-aziridinyl)phosphine sulphide]. Zh. Anal. Khim., 23, 1265-1268

Kaslow, R.A., Wisch, N. & Glass, J.L. (1972) Acute leukaemia following cytostatic therapy. J. Amer. med. Ass., 219, 75-76

Klatt, O., Griffin, A.C. & Stehlin, J.S., Jr (1960) Method for determination of phenylalanine mustard and related alkylating agents in blood. Proc. Soc. exp. Biol. (N.Y.), 104, 629-631

Knipling, E.F., Laven, H., Craig, G.B., Pal, R., Kitzmiller, J.B., Smith, C.N. & Brown, A.W.A. (1968) Genetic control of insects of public health importance. Bull. Wld Hlth Org., 38, 421-438

Krementz, E.T. & Ryan, R.F. (1972) Chemotherapy of melanoma of the extremities by perfusion: fourteen years' clinical experience. Ann. Surg., 175, 900-917

Kuh, E. & Seeger, D.R. (1954) Thiophosphoric acid derivatives. US Patent, 2,670,347, February 23, American Cyanamid Co.

Lidaks, M., Lein, Z. & Shimaskaya, M.V. (1959) The stability of N,N',N''-triethylenethiophosphoramide preparations. Latvijas PSR Zinatnu Akad. Vestis, 11, 87

Lüers, H. & Röhrborn, G. (1965) Chemische Konstitution und mutagene Wirkung. III. Äthylenimine. Mutation Res., 2, 29-44

Machemer, L. & Hess, R. (1971) Comparative dominant lethal studies with phenylbutazone, thio-TEPA and MMS in the mouse. Experientia, 27, 1050-1057

Medical Economics Co. (1974) Physicians' Desk Reference, 28th ed., Oradell, N.J., p. 872

Mellett, L.B. & Woods, L.A. (1960) The comparative physiological disposition of thio-TEPA and TEPA in the dog. Cancer Res., 20, 524-532

Mellett, L.B., Hodgson, P.E. & Woods, L.A. (1962) Absorption and fate of C^{14}-labeled N,N',N''-triethylenethiophosphoramide (thio-TEPA) in humans and dogs. J. Lab. clin. Med., 60, 818-825

Mirkina, N.N. & Kharlamov, V.T. (1965) Thin-layer chromatography analysis of ^{35}S-labelled thio-TEPA. Metody Analiza Radioactivn. Preparatov, Sb. Statei, 155-161

Munson, A.E., Rose, W.C. & Bradley, S.G. (1974) Synergistic lethal action of alkylating agents and sodium pentobarbital in the mouse. Pharmacology, 11, 231-240

Murphy, M.L., Del Moro, A. & Lacon, C. (1958) The comparative effects of five polyfunctional alkylating agents on the rat fetus with additional notes on the chick embryo. Ann. N.Y. Acad. Sci., 68, 762-782

Nangniot, P. (1966) Electrochemical methods for quantitative analysis of pesticide residues. Meded. Rijksfaculteit Landbouwwetensch., 31, 447-473

Nuzhdin, N.I. & Nizhnik, G.V. (1968) Fertilization and embryonic development of rabbits after treatment of spermatozoa in vitro with chemical mutagens. Dokl. Biol. Sci., 181, 419-422

Ozolins, N. & Egerts, V. (1968) Determination of some ethylenimine derivatives. Latv. PSR Zinat. Akad. Vestis, Kim. Ser., 5, 554-559

Patterson, R.S., Boston, M.D., Ford, H.R. & Lofgren, C.S. (1971) Techniques for sterilizing large numbers of mosquitoes. Mosquito News, 31, 85-90

Perlman, M. & Walker, R. (1973) Acute leukaemia following cytotoxic chemotherapy. J. Amer. med. Ass., 224, 250

Plapp, F.W. & Casida, J.E. (1958) Ion-exchange chromatography for hydrolysis products of organophosphate insecticides. Analyt. Chem., 30, 1622-1624

Raine, D.N. (1962) Estimation of thiotepa in urine. J. Pharm. Pharmacol., 14, 614-615

Reeves, W.A., Drake, G.L., Jr, Chance, L.H. & Guthrie, J.D. (1957) Flame retardants for cotton using APO- and APS-THPC resins. Textile Res. J., March, 260-266

Ruffner, B.W. (1974) Androgen role in erythroleukaemia after treatment with alkylating agents. Ann. int. Med., 81, 118-119

Schmähl, D. & Osswald, H. (1970) Experimentelle Untersuchungen über carcinogene Wirkungen von Krebs-Chemotherapeutica und Immunosuppressiva. Arzneimittel-Forsch., 20, 1461-1467

Seawright, J.A., Bowman, M.C. & Patterson, R.S. (1971) Tepa and thiotepa: uptake, persistence and stability induced in pupae and adults of Culex pipiens quinquefasciatus. J. econ. Entomol., 64, 452-455

Shay, H., Zarafonetis, C., Smith, N., Woldow, I. & Sun, D.C.H. (1953) Treatment of leukemia with triethylene thiophosphoramide (thio-TEPA). A.M.A. Arch. int. Med., 92, 628-645

Smith, C.N., LaBrecque, G.C. & Borkovec, A.B. (1964) Insect chemosterilants. In: Smith, R.F. & Mittler, T.E., eds, Annual Review of Entomology, Vol. 9, Palo Alto, California, Annual Reviews Inc., pp. 269-284

Société Suisse de Pharmacie (1973) Index Nominum 1973/74, Zurich

Solomon, R.B. & Firat, D. (1971) Acute leukaemia following treatment with irradiation and alkylating agents. N.Y. State J. Med., 71, 2422-2425

Stecher, P.G., ed. (1968) The Merck Index, 8th ed., Rahway, N.J., Merck & Co., p. 1073

Stoner, G.D., Shimkin, M.B., Kniazeff, A.J., Weisburger, J.H., Weisburger, E.K. & Gori, G.B. (1973) Tests for carcinogenicity of food additives and chemotherapeutic agents by the pulmonary tumor response in strain A mice. Cancer Res., 33, 3069-3085

Sypkens-Smit, G.C. & Meyler, L. (1970) Acute myeloid leukaemia after treatment with cytostatic agents. Lancet, ii, 671-672

Tan, Y.L. & Cole, D.R. (1965) New method for determination of alkylating agents in biologic fluids. Clin. Chem., 11, 58-62

Tanimura, T. (1968) Relation of dosage and time of administration to teratogenic effects of thio-TEPA in mice. Okajimas Folia anat. jap., 44, 203-253

Truhaut, R., Delacoux, E., Brule, G. & Bohuon, C. (1963) Dosage des agents alcoylants dans les milieux biologiques. Méthode utilisant la réaction colorée avec la γ-(nitro-4-benzyl)pyridine en milieu alcalin. Clin. chim. acta, 8, 235-245

US Pharmacopeial Convention Inc. (1970) The US Pharmacopeia, 18th rev., Easton, Pa , Mack, pp. 731-732

White, G.B. (1966) Chemosterilization of Aedes aegypti (L.) by pupal treatment. Nature (Lond.), 210, 1372-1373

Wright, J.C., Golomb, F.M. & Gumport, S.L. (1958) Summary of results with triethylene thiophosphoramide. Ann. N.Y. Acad. Sci., 68, 937-966

94

1. Chemical and Physical Data

1.1 Synonyms and trade names

Chem. Abstr. Reg. Serial No.:   51-18-3

Chem. Abstr. Name: 2,4,6-Tris(1-aziridinyl)-1,3,5-triazine

ENT 25,296; M-9500; R-246; SK-1133; TEM; TET; tretamine; 1,1',1"-s-triazine-2,4,6-triyltrisaziridine; triaziridinyl triazine; triethanomelamine; 2,4,6-triethyleneimino-1,3,5-triazine; triethylene-melamine; 2,4,6-triethylenimino-s-triazine; 2,4,6-tris(1'-aziridinyl)-1,3,5-triazine; 2,4,6-tris(ethyleneimino)-s-triazine; tris(ethylene-imino)triazine; 2,4,6-tris(ethylenimino)-s-triazine

Persistol; Persistol Ho 1/193; Triamelin

1.2 Chemical formula and molecular weight

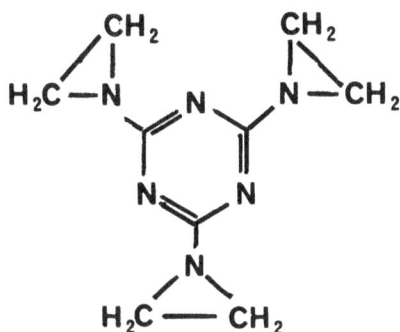

$C_9H_{12}N_6$

Mol. wt: 204.2

1.3 Chemical and physical properties of the pure substance

(a) Description: Colourless crystals from chloroform

(b) Melting-point: 139°C (decomposition); unstable on heating, has no sharp melting-point, although it has been given a melting-point of 150-152°C with decomposition. At 160°C, it initially melts, then rapidly polymerizes to a white solid (Goldenthal et al., 1958).

(c) Spectroscopy data: λ_{max} 226 nm in chloroform is used to identify the compound (Nadkarni et al., 1954). Details of its infrared spectrum are given by Spell (1967).

(d) Solubility: At 26°C the solubility in water was 40%; in chloroform, 28%; in methylene chloride, 20%; in methanol, 12.5%; in acetone, 10.6%; in dioxane, 9.6%; in ethanol, 7.7%; in benzene, 5.6%; in dimethyl cellosolve, 4.9%; in methyl ethyl ketone, 4.7%; in ethyl acetate, 4.5%; in carbon tetrachloride, 3.6% (Wystrach et al., 1955).

(e) Stability: Stable at low temperatures, but polymerizes readily on heating. An aqueous solution can be kept for several months at 4°C in sealed ampoules without appreciable decomposition (Hendry et al., 1951). Studies at 25°C in buffers at pH 7.5, 5.0 and 3.0 showed that there is almost immediate degradation at pH 3.0; even at pH 5.0, degradation was rapid; but at pH 7.5 there was very little degradation even after 24 hours (Beroza & Borkovec, 1964). Recrystallized from chloroform and stored as a solid, it has been found to be stable in air at 5°C or 25°C or under nitrogen at 5°C for at least 48 days; no polymer formation was detected. Storage of the solid at 75°C led to polymerization at a rate of approximately 0.25% per day (Wystrach et al., 1955).

1.4 Technical products and impurities

2,4,6-Tris(1-aziridinyl)-s-triazine (TEM) was available in the US in the form of tablets containing 5 mg (Medical Economics Co., 1974). In Europe it was also available as 5 mg tablets (Bundesverband der Pharmazeutischen Industrie, 1974), as enteric-coated tablets containing 2.5 mg and as ampoules containing 5 mg of the powder (Blacow, 1967).

2. Production, Use, Occurrence and Analysis

For important background information on this section, see preamble, p. 17.

96

2.1 Production and use

TEM can be prepared by the addition of cyanuric chloride to aziridine (Wystrach *et al.*, 1955).

The sole manufacturer of TEM in the US began commercial production in 1954 (Council on Drugs of the American Medical Association, 1963); however, by 1973, less than 1 kg of this chemical was manufactured, and according to the producer its production has been discontinued. In Europe TEM was sold by at least two companies, but it has now been withdrawn from the market. It is believed that TEM has been manufactured in Japan on a laboratory scale for testing as a pharmaceutical intermediate and as a cross-linking agent.

The only known commercial use for TEM in the US was as an antineoplastic agent (Anon., 1959). It was reportedly most effective in the treatment of leukaemias, particularly of chronic lymphocytic leukaemia and chronic myelo-cytic leukaemia, and of malignant lymphomas, especially Hodgkin's disease and lymphosarcoma (Rundles *et al.*, 1958). The recommended dosage was 2.5-5 mg twice weekly, initially for four weeks (Anon., 1972).

TEM has also been used in the manufacture of resinous products and textile finishing agents (Dermer & Ham, 1969), and as a modifier for certain adhesives (Dermer & Hart, 1966).

It has also been tested as an insect chemosterilant (Smith *et al.*, 1964), but it is believed that problems associated with its application to insects, its toxicity and environmental effects have prevented its use in this way on a commercial basis.

2.2 Occurrence

TEM is not known to occur in nature.

2.3 Analysis

TEM can be analysed colorimetrically using 4-(4'-nitrobenzyl)pyridine (Epstein *et al.*, 1955; Preussmann *et al.*, 1969; Truhaut *et al.*, 1963).

The aziridine groups present in TEM can be estimated by using an excess of thiosulphate in an acid solution and back-titrating with base (Beroza & Borkovec, 1964). An alternative titrimetric method has been described by

Schlitt (1963) using potassium thiocyanate in methanol and adding standard *para*-toluenesulphonic acid with methanolic KOH as titrant.

TEM can be separated by thin-layer chromatography, e.g., using a chloroform:acetone solution (1:1), Rf 0.34 (Beroza & Borkovec, 1964). Alternative systems are described by Nadkarni *et al*. (1954) using paper chromatography with either *n*-butanol saturated with 1% ammonia solution or an acetone:water system (3:2 v/v), in which TEM had Rf values of 0.64 and 0.85, respectively. A number of additional solvent systems for paper chromatography and a method for separation by ion-exchange chromatography are described by the same authors in a later paper (Goldenthal *et al*., 1958).

3. Biological Data Relevant to the Evaluation of Carcinogenic Risk to Man

3.1 Carcinogenicity and related studies in animals

(a) Skin application

Mouse: Two groups of 10 male stock albino S mice, 7-9 weeks old, were treated with either a single application of 0.24 mg TEM (as a 0.08% solution in acetone) or 15 weekly applications of a 0.04% solution of TEM (total dose, 1.8 mg); none of the mice developed skin tumours during this treatment. When animals were treated with a single application of 0.24 or 0.5 mg TEM and were also given weekly applications of 0.3 ml of a 0.5% solution of croton oil in acetone for 20 weeks, starting 3 weeks after the application of TEM, 5/10 and 3/7 surviving mice developed a total of 18 and 7 skin papillomas. Fifteen weekly applications of a 0.04% solution of TEM (total dose, 1.8 mg) in conjunction with 22 weekly paintings with croton oil, the first application starting 3 days after the first application of TEM, resulted in the appearance of 22 skin papillomas in 7/10 mice surviving one week after the last application of croton oil. Croton oil alone produced 3 tumours in 1/20 controls. Ten mice treated with TEM and croton oil were examined 22-35 weeks after the croton oil treatment had ended, and 7/10 animals had lung tumours: a total of 63 adenomas were found. Of 15 control mice treated with croton oil alone for up to 72 weeks, 5 had lung tumours, with a total of 27 lung adenomas (Roe & Salaman, 1955).

(b)   Subcutaneous and/or intramuscular administration

Rat: Repeated s.c. injections of TEM in arachis oil into stock rats
(total dose, 10 mg/kg bw) produced local sarcomas in 11/12 treated animals,
with an induction time of 240-450 days.   In an experiment under the same
conditions using inbred Wistar rats, 5/12 rats developed local sarcomas,
with an induction time of 438-506 days;   2 of these animals also developed
hepatomas and 2, ovarian tumours.   No control data were reported (Walpole,
1958).

(c)   Intraperitoneal administration

Mouse: Ten 3-month old male A mice received ten doses of 0.0075 mg
TEM by i.p. injection on alternate days, and surviving animals were killed
100 days after the first injection.   Pulmonary adenomas occurred in 8/10
treated mice, with an average of 2 tumours per mouse.   Of 15 untreated
controls killed at the same time, one had 3 lung tumours and another,
1 lung tumour (Hendry *et al.*, 1951).

Two groups of 9 and 28 virgin female A mice, 3 months old, were given
single i.p. injections of 0.05 mg TEM or two injections of 0.05 mg TEM in
0.1 ml water.   Eighteen weeks after the start of treatment 7/9 animals
given a single injection had pulmonary tumours, with an average of 1.44
tumours/mouse;   in the group given two injections, 24/28 mice developed lung
tumours, with an average of 2.64 tumours/mouse.   The lung tumour incidence
in untreated control females was 3/20 (average, 0.15 tumours/mouse) (Shimkin,
1954).

A group of 113 10-week old female RF mice was given 4 i.p. injections
of 1.5 mg/kg bw TEM in saline at 14-day intervals.   The average survival
time was 427 days, compared with 632 days in controls.   Of 99 treated mice
surviving 30 days or more, 33% developed thymic lymphomas, 53%, pulmonary
adenomas and 52%, ovarian tumours (not specified), compared with 10%, 15%
and 20% in 112 controls, respectively (Conklin *et al.*, 1965).   [These
results were significant ($P<0.001$) for all tumour types: 33/99 *versus*
11/112 for thymic lymphomas, 52/99 *versus* 16/112 for pulmonary adenomas
and 51/99 *versus* 22/112 for ovarian tumours.]

3.2 Other relevant biological data

The i.p. LD$_{50}$ in mice is 4 mg/kg bw (Stecher, 1968).

Following i.p. administration to mice of TEM labelled with ^{14}C in the triazine ring, most of the activity was excreted in urine within 24 hours; the principal metabolite was cyanuric acid (Nadkarni *et al.*, 1954). In mice injected intraperitoneally with 9 mg/kg bw TEM in which the aziridine rings were labelled with ^{14}C, about 70% of the administered radioactivity was excreted in urine within the first 24 hours, and 16 radioactive metabolites were found; only one, creatinine, was identified. Following its i.v. injection in mice at a dose of 0.8 mg/kg bw or in Osborne-Mendel rats at doses of 0.11 and 0.13 mg/kg bw, TEM disappeared rapidly from the blood: within 10 minutes the level had fallen to less than 10% of the original activity (Goldenthal *et al.*, 1958).

Thiersch (1957) found 78% foetal resorption in rats after treatment with two doses of 0.3 mg/kg bw, and 100% resorption with two doses of 0.5 mg/kg bw given on either the 4th and 5th days or the 7th and 8th days of pregnancy. Treatment at a later stage (days 11 and 12 of gestation) resulted in a lower incidence of foetal resorption (16%). TEM produced a decrease in placental weight, and cranial malformations were observed in some surviving foetuses. A single injection of 0.55 mg/kg bw to rats on the 12th day of pregnancy caused 50% foetal resorption, generally ·a decrease in foetal size and characteristic abnormalities such as syndactylous forepaws and some encephaloceles (Murphy *et al.*, 1958).

TEM reacts with the N-7 of guanine in DNA (Tomasz, 1970). It induces point mutations in the purple adenine genes (ad-3A and ad-3B) of *Neurospora crassa* and interstitial deletions of these two loci (Malling & de Serres, 1969). It caused reversions of base-pair substitution mutations in both *Salmonella typhimurium* and *Saccharomyces cerevisiae* (Brusick & Zeiger, 1972) and increased the frequency of sex-linked recessive lethals and chromosomes Y, II and III translocations (Watson, 1964).

TEM induces dominant lethals in male HA/ICR mice (Thayer & Kensler, 1973) and in T-stock, (101xC3H)F$_1$ and (SECxC57BL)F$_1$ female mice (Generoso *et al.*, 1971) after single i.p. injections of 0.02 or 1.6 mg/kg bw.

100

Induction of dominant lethal mutations has also been found to occur after its i.p. injection in male rats (Bateman, 1960) and in male golden hamsters (Lyon & Smith, 1971). A high frequency of transmissible translocations was found among the male and female offspring of male mice injected intraperitoneally with 0.64 mg/kg bw and 0.8 mg/kg bw TEM (Cattanach, 1957). A significant increase in the frequency of morphological specific locus mutations was found among the progeny after i.p. injections of 2 mg/kg bw at 24-hour intervals to parent male (101xC3H)F_1 mice (Cattanach, 1966). TEM also increased the number of histocompatibility mutations in BALB/c and (BALB/cxC57BL/6)F_1 mice after i.p. injection of doses ranging from 2.4-4.0 mg/kg bw (Kohn, 1973).

TEM induces chromosome aberrations in cultured human leucocytes (Hampel *et al.*, 1966).

A patient with acute lymphatic leukaemia was given TEM labelled with ^{14}C in the aziridine ring intravenously at a dose of 2 mg, and, as found in animal studies, over 90% of the radioactivity disappeared from the blood within 5 minutes. In a second cancer patient with metastasizing epidermal carcinoma, 3 mg of the drug were given orally. In both cases 25-30% of the administered activity was excreted in urine collected within the first 48 hours after treatment (Nadkarni *et al.*, 1961). Urine from cancer patients treated with labelled TEM contained 14 radioactive metabolites. Approximately 8% of the radioactivity excreted in the urine was in urea and creatinine; no unchanged drug was detected (Nadkarni *et al.*, 1959).

In a review of the literature Sokal & Lessmann (1960) found three cases in which TEM had been given during pregnancy. Two had Hodgkin's disease and the third a subacute lymphatic leukaemia. Apart from a depressed white cell blood count found in one child at birth, there was no evidence of any adverse effect on the infants at birth in one case nor after 5 or 7 years of age in the other two cases.

3.3 Observations in man

No data were available to the Working Group.

4. Comments on Data Reported and Evaluation[1]

4.1 Animal data

2,4,6-Tris(1-aziridinyl)-s-triazine is carcinogenic in mice following its intraperitoneal injection, producing an increase in the incidence of ovarian, thymic and lung tumours. It also acted as an initiator of skin carcinogenesis. In rats it produced sarcomas at the site of its subcutaneous injection.

4.2 Human data

No case reports or epidemiological studies were available to the Working Group.

---

[1]See also the section, "Animal Data in Relation to the Evaluation of Risk to Man" in the introduction to this volume, p. 15.

5. References

Anon. (1959) Cancer. Chemical and Engineering News, October 12, pp. 53-71

Anon. (1972) Neoplasm therapy. Pharmindex, January, p. 120

Bateman, A.J. (1960) The induction of dominant lethal mutations in rats and mice with triethylenemelamine (TEM). Genet. Res., 1, 381-392

Beroza, M. & Borkovec, A.B. (1964) The stability of tepa and other aziridine chemosterilants. J. med. Chem., 7, 44-49

Blacow, N.W., ed. (1967) Martindale: The Extra Pharmacopoeia, 25th ed., London, The Pharmaceutical Press, pp. 831-832

Brusick, D.J. & Zeiger, E. (1972) A comparison of chemically induced reversion patterns of Salmonella typhimurium and Saccharomyces cerevisiae mutants, using in vitro plate tests. Mutation Res., 14, 271-275

Bundesverband der Pharmazeutischen Industrie (1974) Rote Liste, Aulendorf/ Württ., Editio Cantor

Cattanach, B.M. (1957) Induction of translocations in mice by triethylenemelamine. Nature (Lond.), 180, 1364-1365

Cattanach, B.M. (1966) Chemically induced mutations in mice. Mutation Res., 3, 346-353

Conklin, J.W., Upton, A.C. & Christenberry, K.W. (1965) Further observations on late somatic effects of radiomimetic chemicals and X-rays in mice. Cancer Res., 25, 20-27

Council on Drugs of the American Medical Association (1963) New and Nonofficial Drugs, Philadelphia, Pa , Lippincott, pp. 253-255

Dermer, O.C. & Ham, G.E. (1969) Ethyleneimine and other Aziridines: Chemistry and Applications, New York, Academic Press

Dermer, O.C. & Hart, A.W. (1966) Imines, Cyclic. In: Kirk, R.E. & Othmer, D.F., eds, Encyclopedia of Chemical Technology, 2nd ed., Vol. 11, New York, John Wiley and Sons, pp. 526-548

Epstein, J., Rosenthal, W. & Ess, R.J. (1955) Use of γ-(4-nitrobenzyl)-pyridine as analytical reagent for ethyleneimines and alkylating agents. Analyt. Chem., 27, 1435-1439

Generoso, W.M., Huff, S.W. & Stout, S.K. (1971) Chemically induced dominant-lethal mutations and cell killing in mouse oocytes in the advanced stages of follicular development. Mutation Res., 11, 411-420

Goldenthal, E.I., Nadkarni, M.V. & Smith, P.K. (1958) The excretion of radioactivity following administration of tri-C^{14}-ethylenimino-s-triazine in normal mice. J. Pharmacol. exp. Ther., 122, 431-441

Hampel, K.E., Kober, B., Rösch, D., Gerhartz, H. & Meinig, K.-H. (1966) The action of cytostatic agents on the chromosomes of human leukocytes *in vitro* (preliminary communication). Blood, 27, 816-823

Hendry, J.A., Homer, R.F., Rose, F.L. & Walpole, A.L. (1951) Cytotoxic agents. III. Derivatives of ethyleneimine. Brit. J. Pharmacol., 6, 357-410

Kohn, H.I. (1973) H-gene (histocompatibility) mutations induced by triethylenemelamine in the mouse. Mutation Res., 20, 235-242

Lyon, M.F. & Smith, B.D. (1971) Species comparisons concerning radiation-induced dominant lethals and chromosome aberrations. Mutation Res., 11, 45-58

Malling, H.V. & de Serres, F.J. (1969) Genetic analysis of triethylene melamine induced purple adenine mutants (ad-3) in *Neurospora crassa*. In: Starr, R.C., ed., Proceedings of the International Botanical Conference, NY, Hafner Service, p. 139

Medical Economics Co. (1974) Physicians' Desk Reference, 28th ed., Oradell, N.J., pp. 872-873

Murphy, M.L., Del Moro, A. & Lacon, C. (1958) The comparative effects of five polyfunctional alkylating agents on the rat fetus, with additional notes on the chick embryo. Ann. N.Y. Acad. Sci., 68, 762-782

Nadkarni, M.V., Goldenthal, E.I. & Smith, P.K. (1954) The distribution of radioactivity following administration of triethylenimino-s-triazine-C^{14} in tumor-bearing and control mice. Cancer Res., 14, 559-562

Nadkarni, M.V., Trams, E.G. & Smith, P.K. (1959) Preliminary studies on the distribution and fate of TEM, TEPA and myleran in the human. Cancer Res., 19, 713-718

Nadkarni, M.V., Trams, E.G. & Smith, P.K. (1961) Excretion and distribution studies with radioisotope-labeled alkylating drugs in cancer patients. Cancer, 14, 953-956

Preussmann, R., Schneider, H. & Epple, F. (1969) Untersuchungen zum Nachweis alkylierender Agentien. II. Der Nachweis verschiedener Klassen alkylierender Agentien mit einer Modifikation der Farbreaktion mit 4-(4-Nitrobenzyl)pyridin (NBP). Arzneimittel-Forsch., 19, 1059-1073

Roe, F.J.C. & Salaman, M.H. (1955) Further studies on incomplete carcinogenesis: triethylene melamine (TEM), 1,2-benzanthracene and β-propiolactone as initiators of skin tumour formation in the mouse. Brit. J. Cancer, 9, 177-203

Rundles, R.W., Coonrad, E.V. & Willard, N.L. (1958) Summary of results obtained with TEM. Ann. N.Y. Acad. Sci., 68, 926-936

Schlitt, R.C. (1963) Assay of aziridinyl compounds. Analyt. Chem., 35, 1063-1064

Shimkin, M.B. (1954) Pulmonary tumor induction in mice with chemical agents used in the clinical management of lymphomas. Cancer, 7, 410-413

Smith, C.N., LaBrecque, G.C. & Borkovec, A.B. (1964) Insect Chemosterilants. In: Smith, R.F. & Mittler, T.E., eds, Annual Review of Entomology, Vol. 9, Palo Alto, California, Annual Reviews Inc., pp. 269-284

Sokal, J.E. & Lessmann, E.M. (1960) Effects of cancer chemotherapeutic agents on the human fetus. J. Amer. med. Ass., 172, 1765-1771

Spell, H.L. (1967) The infrared spectra of N-substituted aziridine compounds. Analyt. Chem., 39, 185-193

Stecher, P.G., ed. (1968) The Merck Index, 8th ed., Rahway, N.J., Merck & Co., p. 1073

Thayer, P.S. & Kensler, C.J. (1973) Genetic tests in mice of caffeine alone and in combination with mutagens. Toxicol. appl. Pharmacol., 25, 157-168

Thiersch, J.B. (1957) Effect of 2,4,6-triamino-"S"-triazine (TR), 2,4,6-"tris"(ethylenimino)-"S"-triazine (TEM) and N,N',N''-triethylenephosphoramide (TEPA) on rat litter in $utero$. Proc. Soc. exp. Biol. (N.Y.), 94, 36-40

Tomasz, M. (1970) Novel assay of 7-alkylation of guanine residues in DNA application to nitrogen mustard, triethylenemelamine and mitomycin C. Biochim. biophys. acta, 213, 288-295

Truhaut, R., Delacoux, E., Brule, G. & Bohuon, C. (1963) Dosage des agents alcoylants dans les milieux biologiques. Méthode utilisant la réaction colorée avec la γ-(nitro-4-benzyl)-pyridine en milieu alcalin. Clin. chim. acta, 8, 235-245

Walpole, A.L. (1958) Carcinogenic action of alkylating agents. Ann. N.Y. Acad. Sci., 68, 750-761

Watson, W.A.F. (1964) Evidence of an essential difference between the genetical effects of mono- and bi-functional alkylating agents. Z. Vererbungsl., 95, 374-378

Wystrach, V.P., Kaiser, D.W. & Schaefer, F.C. (1955) Preparation of ethylenimine and triethylenemelamine. J. Amer. chem. Soc., 77, 5915-5918

TRIS(2-METHYL-1-AZIRIDINYL)PHOSPHINE OXIDE

1. Chemical and Physical Data

1.1 Synonyms and trade names

Chem. Abstr. Reg. Serial No.:   57-39-6

Chem. Abstr. Name: 1,1'1"-Phosphinylidynetris(2-methyl)aziridine

EMT 50,003; MAPO; metapoxide; metepa; methaphoxide; methyl aphoxide; tris(methylaziridinyl)phosphine oxide; tris(methyl-1-aziridinyl)phosphine oxide; tris(2-methylaziridin-1-yl)phosphine oxide; N,N',N''-tris(1-methylethylene)phosphoramide; tris(1-methylethylene)phosphoric triamide

1.2 Chemical formula and molecular weight

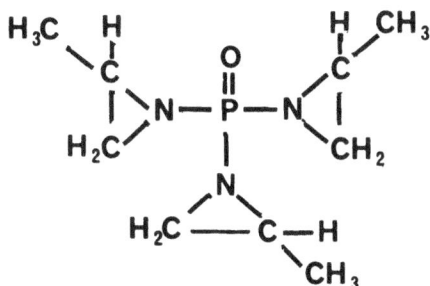

$C_9H_{18}N_3OP$

Mol. wt: 215.2

1.3 Chemical and physical properties of the pure substance

(a) Description: Amber-coloured liquid

(b) Boiling-point: 90-92°C at 0.3 mm Hg;   118°C at 1 mm Hg

(c) Density: d_4^{25} 1.079

(d) Refractive index: n_D^{25} 1.48

(e) Solubility: Miscible with water and organic solvents

(f) Stability: Stable in alkaline solutions, e.g., the time for 50% hydrolysis in 1 N alkali is >100 hours. However, in acid solution it is unstable and is rapidly destroyed. Even at a pH of 5.5-6.0 $t_{\frac{1}{2}}$ is about 6 hours, the main product being phosphoric acid (Plapp et $al.$, 1962). A 0.3% aqueous solution at pH 7.05 will decompose slowly ($t_{\frac{1}{2}}$, >200 days at $3^{O}C$, 72 days at $25^{O}C$, 16.5 days at $50^{O}C$ and <0.1 days at $100^{O}C$) (Beroza & Borkovec, 1964).

1.4 Technical products and impurities

Tris(2-methyl-1-aziridinyl)phosphine oxide (metepa) is available commercially in the United States in quart, and in 1-, 5- and 55-gallon containers. Commercial material contains a minimum of 92% metepa, as determined by a reactive imine assay, and no more than 0.5% volatile material (Anon., undated).

2. Production, Use, Occurrence and Analysis

For important background information on this section, see preamble, p.

2.1 Production and use

Metepa can be synthesized by the addition of phosphorous oxychloride to 2-methylethyleneimine in alkaline medium (Parker et $al.$, 1952).

A US producer first reported commercial production of this chemical in 1961 (US Tariff Commission, 1962), and in 1972 two manufacturers reported production of an unpublished quantity (US Tariff Commission, 1974). Metepa is produced by one French company (Chemical Information Services, Ltd, 1975) and is sold for use as a cross-linking agent.

Metepa is apparently used in the US exclusively as an intermediate, as a cross-linking agent for paint, textile and adhesive polymers containing active hydrogen sites (such as carboxyl, phenol, sulphhydryl, amide and hydroxyl groups). Other possible uses are as a cross-linking agent for textile pigment print systems, rubber, plastics and wash-and-wear cotton clothing (Anon., undated).

Metepa is an effective insect chemosterilant (Borkovec et $al.$, 1968; Keiser et $al.$, 1965; Ouye et $al.$, 1965; Smith et $al.$, 1964; Toppozada et $al.$, 1966), but it is believed that problems associated with its application to insects, its toxicity and environmental effects have prevented its use in this way on a commercial basis.

108

Metepa has also been tested as an antineoplastic agent (Goodridge *et al.*, 1963), but it is probably not used for this purpose.

2.2 Occurrence

Metepa is not known to occur in nature.

2.3 Analysis

Gas chromatographic procedures capable of detecting 1 ng have been developed (Bowman & Beroza, 1966, 1970), based on the use of a flame-photometric detector, which is highly sensitive to phosphorous-containing compounds. This type of analysis is particularly useful in biological experiments: for instance, a simple methanol extract of insect tissue can be assayed directly, without preliminary purification.

Other less sensitive analytical procedures include the reaction of aziridine groups with thiosulphate in acid solution and back-titrating with base. A method using a potassium thiocyanate:*para*-toluenesulphonic acid solution to open the aziridine ring has been described (Schlitt, 1963); it is claimed to be faster and more easily performed than that using thiosulphate. Samples containing metepa have also been assayed in chloroform with standard perchloric acid in the presence of an excess of tetra-butylammonium iodide (Jay, 1964).

A thin-layer chromatographic separation system has been developed, applicable to the separation of metepa and its intermediates, using silica gel plates, in which the spots are detected colorimetrically using a system selective for aziridines. NMR spectrometry for analysis and a colorimetric method for the microdetection of metepa in column eluates (limit, 5 µg) are also described (Beroza & Borkovec, 1964). Metepa can be separated from phosphoric acid and the di- or mono-acid intermediates by solvent partition (Plapp *et al.*, 1962).

3. Biological Data Relevant to the Evaluation of Carcinogenic Risk to Man

3.1 Carcinogenicity and related studies in animals

Oral administration

Rat: Three groups of 20 male Sherman rats, 5-6 weeks of age, were given metepa in water by gavage in doses of 0.625, 2.5 and 5.0 mg/kg bw/day for 422, 422 and 155 days. After 422 days, 15 controls and 19, 9 and 8 treated rats were still alive in the respective dosage groups. Three lymphatic leukaemias occurred in the group given 2.5 mg/kg bw/day; and in the group given 5 mg/kg bw/day, 2 lymphatic leukaemias, 1 chloroleukaemia and 1 astrocytoma occurred. The first animal to develop leukaemia was 7 months old at the time of death. Tumours in the control and lowest dose groups were not reported; the spontaneous tumour incidence in this colony was reported to be low (Gaines & Kimbrough, 1966).

3.2 Other relevant biological data

The oral LD_{50}'s in male and female rats were reported to be 136 and 213 mg/kg bw (Gaines, 1969). The no-effect level in male rats over 84 days was 2.5 mg/kg bw/day given by stomach tube. In mice, the oral LD_{50} was 292 mg/kg bw, the LD_{50} following skin application, 375 mg/kg bw and the s.c. LD_{50}, 140 mg/kg bw (Maehashi, 1970).

Two male white mice were injected intraperitoneally with 100 mg/kg bw ^{32}P-metepa. Unchanged metepa was found as the major radioactive component in the blood during the first 2 hours after treatment but had almost disappeared after 6 hours. More than half of the radioactivity was excreted in the urine in the first 12 hours after treatment: unchanged metepa and phosphoric acid were the principal labelled components. The mice died 5-8 days after injection (Plapp *et al.*, 1962).

Six female rats of the Sherman strain were injected intraperitoneally with 30 mg/kg bw metepa on the 12th day of pregnancy. Forty of the foetuses were resorbed, and 16/43 foetuses were born dead. All the neonates (27 alive and 16 dead) had malformations, ectrodactylia being found in all offspring; average birth and placental weights were significantly reduced. In a separate experiment, daily i.p. injections of 1.25 mg/kg bw given on days 7-13 of pregnancy caused a significant reduction in foetal and placental weights. In males, metepa had a sterilizing effect (Gaines & Kimbrough, 1966).

Treatment of male mice with 0.156-20 mg/kg bw metepa resulted in a high frequency of dominant lethals (Epstein *et al*., 1970).

3.3 Observations in man

No data were available to the Working Group.

4. Comments on Data Reported and Evaluation

4.1 Animal data

In the only available study, tris(2-methyl-1-aziridinyl)phosphine oxide was reported to have induced leukaemia in rats following its oral adminis-tration. The data are insufficient for evelution of its carcinogenicity.

4.2 Human data

No case reports or epidemiological studies were available to the Working Group.

5. References

Anon. (undated) _Organic Chemicals: MAPO_, Carlstadt, N.J., Arsynco Inc.

Beroza, M. & Borkovec, A.B. (1964) The stability of tepa and other aziridine chemosterilants. _J. med. Chem._, _7_, 44-49

Borkovec, A.B., Nagasawa, S. & Shinohara, H. (1968) Sterilization of the azuki bean weevil, _Callosobruchus Chinensis_, by metepa and hempa. _J. econ. Entomol._, _61_, 695-698

Bowman, M.C. & Beroza, M. (1966) Gas chromatographic determination of trace amounts of the insect chemosterilants tepa, metepa, methiotepa, hempa and apholate and the analysis of tepa in insect tissue. _J. Ass. off. analyt. Chem._, _49_, 1046-1052

Bowman, M.C. & Beroza, M. (1970) GLC retention times of pesticides and metabolites containing phosphorus and sulphur on four thermally stable columns. _J. Ass. off. analyt. Chem._, _53_, 499-508

Chemical Information Services, Ltd. (1975) _Directory of Western European Chemical Producers_, 1975/76, Oceanside, NY

Epstein, S.S., Arnold, E., Steinberg, K., Mackintosh, D., Shafner, H. & Bishop, Y. (1970) Mutagenic and antifertility effects of TEPA and METEPA in mice. _Toxicol. appl. Pharmacol._, _17_, 23-40

Gaines, T.B. (1969) Acute toxicity of pesticides. _Toxicol. appl. Pharmacol._, _14_, 515-534

Gaines, T.B. & Kimbrough, R.D. (1966) The sterilising, carcinogenic and teratogenic effects of metepa in rats. _Bull. Wld Hlth Org._, _34_, 317-320

Goodridge, T.H., Huntress, W.T. & Bratzel, R.P. (1963) Survey of aziridines. _Cancer Chemother. Rep._, _26_, 434

Jay, R.R. (1964) Direct titration of epoxy compounds and aziridines. _Analyt. Chem._, _36_, 667-668

Keiser, I., Steiner, L.F. & Kamasaki, H. (1965) Effect of chemosterilants against the oriental fruit fly, melon fly and Mediterranean fruit fly. _J. econ. Entomol._, _58_, 682-685

Maehashi, H. (1970) Toxicity of chemosterilants. I. Toxicity of alkylating agent 'metepa' to rats and mice. _Ind. Hlth (Jap.)_, _84_, 54-65

Ouye, M.T., Grahamm, H.M., Garcia, R.S. & Martin, D.F. (1965) Comparative mating competitiveness of metepa-sterilized and normal pink bollworm males in laboratory and field cages. _J. econ. Entomol._, _58_, 927-929

Parker, R.P., Seeger, D.R. & Kuh, E. (1952) US Patent, 2,606,900, August 12, American Cyanamid Co.

Plapp, F.W., Jr, Bigley, W.S., Chapman, G.A. & Eddy, G.W. (1962) Metabolism of methaphoxide in mosquitoes, house flies and mice. J. econ. Entomol., 55, 607-613

Schlitt, R.C. (1963) Assay of aziridinyl compounds. Analyt. Chem., 35, 1063-1064

Smith, C.N., LaBrecque, G.C. & Borkovec, A.B. (1964) Insect Chemosterilants. In: Smith, R.F. & Mittler, T.E., eds, Annual Review of Entomology, Vol. 9, Palo Alto, California, Annual Reviews Inc., pp. 269-283

Toppozada, A., Abdullah, S. & Eldefrawi, M.E. (1966) Chemosterilisation of larvae and adults of the Egyptian cotton leafworm, *Prodenia litura*, by apholate, metepa and tepa. J. econ. Entomol., 59, 1125-1128

US Tariff Commission (1962) Synthetic Organic Chemicals, US Production and Sales, 1961, TC Publication 72, Washington DC, US Government Printing Office, p. 86

US Tariff Commission (1974) Synthetic Organic Chemicals, US Production and Sales, 1972, TC Publication 681, Washington DC, US Government Printing Office, p. 52

MUSTARDS

BIS(2-CHLOROETHYL)ETHER

1. Chemical and Physical Data

1.1 Synonyms and trade names

Chem. Abstr. Reg. Serial No.:   111-44-4

Chem. Abstr. Name: 1,1'-Oxybis(2-chloro)ethane

Bis(chloroethyl)ether; bis(β-chloroethyl)ether; 1-chloro-2-(β-chloroethoxy)ethane; DCEE; 2,2'-dichlorodiethyl ether; β,β'-dichlorodiethyl ether; dichloroether; dichloroethyl ether; 2,2'-dichloroethyl ether; β,β'-dichloroethyl ether; di-2-chloroethyl ether; di(2-chloroethyl)ether; di(β-chloroethyl)ether; dichloroethyl oxide; sym-dichloroethyl ether

Chlorex

1.2 Chemical formula and molecular weight

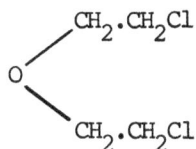

$$O \Big\langle \begin{array}{l} CH_2.CH_2Cl \\ CH_2.CH_2Cl \end{array}$$

$C_4H_8Cl_2O$ Mol. wt: 143

1.3 Chemical and physical properties of the pure substance

(a) Description: A colourless, non-flammable liquid

(b) Boiling-point: 176-178°C at 760 mm Hg;   66°C at 12 mm Hg; 70°C at 15 mm Hg;   82-83°C at 23 mm Hg

(c) Melting-point: -24.5°C

(d) Density: d_4^{20} 1.213

(e) Refractive index: n_D^{20} 1.457

(f) Solubility: Miscible with most organic solvents;   insoluble in water

(g) Volatility: Low volatility

(h) <u>Stability</u>:   Hydrolysed slowly in aqueous dimethylformamide at pH 7 (K_W 30°C <5.0x10^{-4} min^{-1})

1.4   Technical products and impurities

Bis(2-chloroethyl)ether has been available in the United States in technical and purified grades. Typical specifications for the compound limit the maximum percentage by weight of acidity (as HCl) to 0.005% and of water to 0.10% (Lurie, 1965). It has been marketed as an emulsifiable concentrate and an aerosol as an ingredient of pesticide products: the concentrate has been reported to contain 70% bis(2-chloroethyl)ether and copper chloride (1% metallic copper); the aerosol has been reported to contain 1.25% bis(2-chloroethyl)ether formulated with β-butoxy-β'-thiocyano diethyl ether and pine oil (US Environmental Protection Agency, 1974a).

2.   Production, Use, Occurrence and Analysis

For important background information on this section, see preamble, p. 17.

2.1 Production and use

Bis(2-chloroethyl)ether can be prepared by treating ethylene chloro-hydrin with sulphuric acids; by saturating an aqueous solution of ethylene chlorohydrin with chlorine and ethylene; or by chlorinating diethyl ether (Lurie, 1965; Martin, 1971). Bis(2-chloroethyl)ether was prepared commercially in the US as a by-product in the manufacture of ethylene oxide by the chlorohydrin process.

According to industry sources, approximately 1.8 million kg of the chemical were sold by one US company in 1973; however, since the company discontinued use of the chlorohydrin process at that time, bis(2-chloro-ethyl)ether is no longer produced for sale in the US in commercial quantities. Two US companies produce bis(2-chloroethyl)ether for use within their own plants and among subsidiaries. One of these companies produces less than 0.5 million kg annually for use as a solvent and as a chemical intermediate in proprietary processes. Two US companies have recently investigated the feasibility of future production of the chemical. Bis(2-chloroethyl)ether is produced in commercial quantities by one company in Japan; however, production volume and trade data have not been reported. This chemical is also manufactured in the Federal Republic of Germany (Chemical Information Services, Ltd, 1975).

Bis(2-chloroethyl)ether has been used as a soil fumigant, as an insecticide and as an acaricide (Anon., 1975; US Environmental Protection Agency, 1974a). It has also been used as a solvent for fats, waxes, greases and cellulose esters; as a scouring agent for textiles (Lurie, 1965); in paints, varnishes and lacquers; as a paint remover; in dry cleaning (Hawley, 1971); and has been reportedly used as an intermediate in the synthesis of morpholine and N-substituted morpholine compounds and of divinyl ether, an anaesthetic. It can be used to scavenge lead deposits in gasoline but apparently has never found commercial use in this way.

2.2 Occurrence

Analysis of New Orleans' drinking-water confirmed the presence of bis(2-chloroethyl)ether at three different plant sites in concentrations of 0.7, 0.12 and 0.16 µg/l (US Environmental Protection Agency, 1974b). It is believed that chlorine, added to purify the drinking-water, may react with hydrocarbons present in the water to form chlorinated derivatives, such as bis(2-chloroethyl)ether (Marx, 1974).

2.3 Analysis

Gas chromatographic methods have been developed for the determination of 34 fumigants, including bis(2-chloroethyl)ether, with a detection limit of 1 µg (Berck, 1965). Bis(2-chloroethyl)ether has been determined in air by a colorimetric reaction with quinoline (detection limit, 2 µg/l) or with pyridine and alkali in the presence of amines (detection limit, 0.5 µg/l) (Tupeeva, 1969).

3. Biological Data Relevant to the Evaluation of Carcinogenic Risk to Man

3.1 Carcinogenicity and related studies in animals

(a) Oral administration

Mouse: Two groups of 18 male and 18 female mice of the (C57Bl/6x C3H/Anf)F_1 or (C57Bl/6xAKR)F_1 strain were given the same absolute amount of 100 mg/kg bw bis(2-chloroethyl)ether by stomach tube daily from the 7th to 28th day of age. Subsequently, the chemical was fed at a concentration of 300 mg/kg bw in the diet for 80 weeks. Of the (C57Bl/6xC3H/Anf)F_1 mice, 14/16 males developed hepatomas and 2/16, lymphomas; and 4/18 females developed hepatomas. Of the (C57Bl/6xAKR)F_1 mice, 9/17 males developed hepatomas and 2/17, pulmonary adenomas; only 1 lymphoma was observed among 18 females. The incidences of hepatomas in male and female controls of the two strains were 8/79 and 0/87 in (C57Bl/6xC3H/Anf)F_1 mice and 5/90 and 1/82 in (C57Bl/6xAKR)F_1 mice. The incidence of hepatomas in male treated mice compared with that in controls was significantly different at the P=0.01 level (Innes *et al.*, 1969; National Technical Information Service, 1968).

(b) Skin application

Mouse: A group of 20 female ICR/Ha Swiss mice, 6 weeks of age, was given the highest dose possible with minimal cytotoxic effects (1 mg in 0.1 ml benzene) once; then the tumour promotor, phorbol myristate acetate, was given at 2.5 µg in 100 µl acetone thrice weekly starting 14 days after the primary treatment (median survival time, 459 days). Three mice developed papillomas within 604 days, compared with 2/20 controls given phorbol myristate acetate alone (Van Duuren *et al.*, 1972). [P>0.05].

(c) Subcutaneous and/or intramuscular administration

Mouse: A group of 30 female ICR/Ha Swiss mice, 6 weeks of age, was given weekly s.c. injections of 1 mg bis(2-chloroethyl)ether in 0.05 ml purified paraffin oil for life (median survival time, 656 days). Within 685 days 2 mice had developed sarcomas at the injection site. No tumours occurred in 30 controls given 0.05 ml purified paraffin oil alone (mean survival time, 643 days) (Van Duuren *et al.*, 1972). [P>0.05].

3.2 Other relevant biological data

Acute toxic amounts of the compound rapidly penetrated the skin of rabbits and caused death within one day (Smyth & Carpenter, 1948). The single-dose oral LD_{50} for rats has been reported as 75 mg/kg bw (Smyth & Carpenter, 1948), 105 mg/kg bw (Spector, 1956) or 150 mg/kg bw (Hake & Rowe, 1967), and for mice and rabbits, 136 mg/kg bw and 126 mg/kg bw, respectively (Spector, 1956). Guinea-pigs exposed to continuous inhalation of 500-1000 ppm in air died after 5-8 hours from respiratory injuries (Schrenk *et al.*, 1933).

Bis(2-chloroethyl)ether vaporizes to an irritant gas. Brief exposures to concentrations above 550 ppm in the air were irritating to the eyes and nasal passages of human volunteers and were considered intolerable. They also caused coughing, retching and nausea (Schrenk *et al.*, 1933).

3.3 Observations in man

No data were available to the Working Group.

4. Comments on Data Reported and Evaluation[1]

4.1 Animal data

Bis(2-chloroethyl)ether produced an increased incidence of liver-cell tumours in male mice of two strains following its oral administration. Its administration by the subcutaneous route in mice produced a low incidence of sarcomas at the injection site.

4.2 Human data

No case reports or epidemiological studies were available to the Working Group.

---

[1]See also the section, "Animal Data in Relation to the Evaluation of Risk to Man" in the introduction to this volume, p. 15.

5. References

Anon. (1975) Farm Chemicals Handbook, Willoughby, Ohio, Meister Publishing Company, p. D68

Berck, B. (1965) Determination of fumigant gases by gas chromatography. J. agric. Fd Chem., 13, 373-377

Chemical Information Services, Ltd (1975) Directory of Western European Chemical Producers, 1975/76, Oceanside, NY

Hake, C.L. & Rowe, V.K. (1967) Ethers. In: Patty, F.A., ed., Industrial Hygiene and Toxicology, 2nd ed., Vol. II, New York, John Wiley and Sons, pp. 1673-1677

Hawley, G.G. (1971) The Condensed Chemical Dictionary, 8th ed., New York, Van Nostrand Reinhold Company, pp. 285-286

Innes, J.R.M., Ulland, B.M., Valerio, M.G., Petrucelli, L., Fishbein, L., Hart, E.R., Pallotta, A.J., Bates, R.R., Falk, H.L., Gart, J.J., Klein, M., Mitchell, I. & Peters, J. (1969) Bioassay of pesticides and industrial chemicals for tumorigenicity in mice: A preliminary report. J. nat. Cancer Inst., 42, 1101-1114

Lurie, A.P. (1965) Ethers. In: Kirk, R.E. & Othmer, D.F., eds, Encyclopedia of Chemical Technology, 2nd ed., Vol. 8, New York, John Wiley and Sons, pp. 486-487

Martin, H., ed. (1971) Pesticide Manual, 2nd ed., Worcester, British Crop Protection Council, p. 161

Marx, J.L. (1974) Drinking water: another source of carcinogens? Science, 186, 809-811

National Technical Information Service (1968) Evaluation of Carcinogenic, Teratogenic and Mutagenic Activities of Selected Pesticides and Industrial Chemicals, Vol. 1, Carcinogenic Study, Washington DC, US Department of Commerce

Schrenk, H.H., Patty, F.A. & Yaut, W.P. (1933) Acute response of guinea pigs to vapors of some new commercial organic compounds. Publ. Hlth Rep. (Wash.), 48, 1389-1397

Smyth, H.F., Jr & Carpenter, C.P. (1948) Further experience with the range finding test in the industrial toxicology laboratory. J. industr. Hyg. Toxicol., 30, 63-68

Spector, W.S., ed. (1956) Handbook of Toxicology, Vol. 1, Philadelphia, Saunders

Tupeeva, R.B. (1969) Separate determination of tetrachloroethylene and β,β'-dichlorodiethyl ether in the air. Tr. Ufim. Nauch.-Issled. Inst. Gig. Prof. Zabol., 5, 239-241

US Environmental Protection Agency (1974a) EPA Compendium of Registered Pesticides, Vol. III, March 29, Washington DC, US Government Printing Office, pp. D-15.1-D-15.2

US Environmental Protection Agency (1974b) Draft Analytical Report, New Orleans Area Water Supply Study, November, Dallas, Texas, p. 22

Van Duuren, B.L., Katz, C., Goldschmidt, B.M., Frenkel, K. & Sivak, A. (1972) Carcinogenicity of halo-ethers. II. Structure-activity relationships of analogs of bis(chloromethyl)ether. J. nat. Cancer Inst., 48, 1431-1439

CHLORAMBUCIL

1. Chemical and Physical Data

1.1 Synonyms and trade names

Chem. Abstr. Reg. Serial No.:   305-03-3

Chem. Abstr. Name: 4-[Bis(2-chloroethyl)amino]benzenebutanoic acid

4-[*para*-Bis(2-chloroethyl)aminophenyl]butyric acid;   4-[*para*-bis(β-chloroethyl)aminophenyl]butyric acid;   γ-[*para*-bis(2-chloroethyl)-aminophenyl]butyric acid;   CB 1348;   chlorobutin;   chlorobutine;   γ-[*para*-di(2-chloroethyl)aminophenyl]butyric acid;   *para*-[di(2-chloro-ethyl)aminophenyl]butyric acid;   *para*-(*N*,*N*-di-2-chloroethyl)amino-phenyl butyric acid;   *N*,*N*-di-2-chloroethyl-γ-*para*-aminophenyl butyric acid;   *para*-*N*,*N*-di(β-chloroethyl)aminophenyl butyric acid;   NSC-3088;   phenylbutyric acid nitrogen mustard

Ambochlorin;   Chloraminophen;   Chloraminophene;   Elcoril;   Leukeran;   Leukersan;   Linfolysin

1.2 Chemical formula and molecular weight

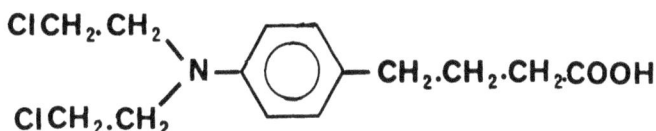

$C_{14}H_{19}Cl_2NO_2$ Mol. wt: 304.2

1.3 Chemical and physical properties of the pure substance

(a) Description: Fine white crystals with slight odour

(b) Melting-point: 64-67°C

(c) Spectroscopy data: A 30 μg/ml ethanolic solution of chlorambucil has a maximal optical density of 1.85 at 258 nm;   in aqueous solution at pH 7 or more, a 30 μg/ml solution of the sodium salt has a maximal optical density of 1.55 at 256 nm (Linford, 1961, 1962).

125

(d) Solubility: The free acid is soluble at 20°C in 1.5 parts ethanol, 2 parts acetone, 2.5 parts chloroform and 2 parts ethyl acetate (British Pharmaceutical Codex, 1973); soluble in benzene and ether. Insoluble in water, but readily soluble in acid or alkali. The sodium salt is soluble in water (Linford, 1961).

(e) Stability: Aqueous solutions of the sodium salt undergo alkali-catalysed hydrolysis to the hydroxyl form, the reaction requiring 30 minutes at 37°C and pH 11.5; no appreciable hydrolysis takes place within 24 hours at 5°C (Linford, 1961).

(f) Reactivity: Hydrolysis in aqueous and alkaline solution leads to replacement of the chlorine atoms by OH groups to give the so-called hydroxyl form (Linford, 1961).

1.4 Technical products and impurities

Chlorambucil is available in USP grade in the form of tablets containing 2 and 5 mg active ingredient (Bundesverband der pharmazeutischen Industrie, 1969; Dictionnaire Vidal, 1975; Kastrup, 1974; Pullom, 1968-69; Steinböck et al., 1969). Chlorambucil powder, USP, used to formulate the tablets, contains 98-101% chlorambucil, calculated on the anhydrous basis. Chlorambucil tablets, USP, contain 93-107% of the labelled amount of chlorambucil (US Pharmacopeial Convention, Inc., 1970).

2. Production, Use, Occurrence and Analysis

For important background information on this section, see preamble, p. 17.

2.1 Production and use

Chlorambucil can be prepared by hydrogenating the methyl or ethyl ester of 4-(para-nitrophenyl)butyric acid in the presence of a catalyst. The resulting para-amino analogue is treated with ethylene oxide followed by chlorination. The resulting 4-[para-bis-2-(chloroethylamino)phenyl]butyric acid ester is converted to the free acid by hydrolysis with hydrochloric acid (Everett et al., 1953).

126

Although chlorambucil tablets have been formulated and marketed in the US by one company since 1957, all chlorambucil used in the US is imported from the United Kingdom. Data on the quantity of imports are not available, but it is estimated that total US sales of this chemical amount to less than 20 kg annually. Chlorambucil is also produced in Italy (Chemical Information Services, Ltd, 1975).

It is used in human medicine as an antineoplastic agent in the treatment of malignant diseases such as lymphocytic leukaemia, malignant lymphomas (including lymphosarcoma), giant follicular lymphoma and Hodgkin's disease. The drug is administered orally in doses of 0.1-0.2 mg/kg bw daily for 3-6 weeks (Huff, 1974). It has also been tested for use in immunosuppressive therapy of chronic hepatitis (Phlippen *et al.*, 1969) and of rheumatoid arthritis (Baum & Vaughan, 1969).

Veterinary uses of chlorambucil are reported to include treatment of leukaemias and, to a lesser degree, of solid tissue tumours (Stecher, 1968).

It has also been investigated as an insect chemosterilant.

2.2 Occurrence

Chlorambucil is not known to occur in nature.

2.3 Analysis

Chlorambucil has been determined in blood by a spectrophotometric method based on its reaction with 4-(4'-nitrobenzyl)pyridine (Boyland *et al.*, 1961). A similar reaction can be applied for determinations in various biological fluids and is sensitive at 5 μg/ml. Kozlov & Bernshtein (1968) detected chlorambucil at concentrations greater than 3 μg/ml in saline solution by reaction with nicotinic acid and benzidine. The substance can also be determined in serum or plasma at 2 μg/ml by direct spectrophotometric measurement (Linford, 1962). The pure drug may be assayed by a titration method (British Pharmacopoeia Commission, 1973).

3. Biological Data Relevant to the Evaluation of Carcinogenic Risk to Man

3.1 Carcinogenicity and related studies in animals

(a) Skin application

Mouse: A group of 25 S mice received 10 weekly skin applications of chlorambucil, 8 at 0.1% and 2 at 0.05% in methanol (total dose, 2.7 mg). Thirty days after the start of treatment the mice were painted once weekly for 18 weeks with croton oil. When the treatments overlapped chlorambucil and croton oil were applied alternately at 3-4 day intervals. Sixty control mice received 18 weekly applications of 0.085-0.5% croton oil. At the end of the treatment 11/19 (58%) mice had developed 30 papillomas (2.7 tumours/mouse), compared with 5/53 controls (1.4 tumours/mouse) [$P<0.001$]; 7/12 mice had developed 13 pulmonary adenomas (1.9 tumours/mouse), but this incidence was not statistically higher than that in controls. No malignant tumours developed in the 6 treated mice kept for longer periods (Salaman & Roe, 1956).

(b) Intraperitoneal administration

Mouse: Groups of 45-60 A/J mice of both sexes, 4-6 weeks old, received i.p. injections of chlorambucil in a 1% acacia solution or in tricaprylin thrice weekly for 4 weeks (total doses, 9.6, 37, 150 and 420 mg/kg bw). At 39 weeks the numbers of survivors were 38/45, 56/60, 47/60 and 30/60, and of these 18 (47%), 48 (86%), 45 (96%) and 30 (100%) had lung tumours (adenomas and adenocarcinomas); there were 0.6, 1.6, 5.1 and 8.9 tumours per mouse, respectively. In 385 male and 392 female controls receiving vehicles only, 39.5% male and 31.4% female survivors developed lung tumours within 39 weeks, the numbers of tumours per mouse being 0.5 and 0.36. The potency of chlorambucil was reported to be about 1/60th that of uracil mustard on a molar basis (Shimkin *et al.*, 1966).

Two groups of 25 male and 25 female Swiss mice, 6 weeks of age, were given i.p. injections of 1.5 or 3 mg/kg bw thrice weekly for 6 months, followed by observation for a further 12 months, at which time the animals were killed. Lung tumours occurred in 22/35 males and in 20/28 females. Lymphosarcomas were found in 6/35 males and 4/28 females, and ovarian tumours

were found in 10/28 females. In each case the incidence for each tumour
type was reported to be significantly different from that in controls
(P<0.01 - P<0.001) (Weisburger *et al.*, 1975).

Rat: Two groups of 25 male and 25 female Charles River CD rats, 6
weeks of age, were given i.p. injections of 2.2 or 4.5 mg/kg bw thrice
weekly for 6 months, followed by observation for a further 12 months, at
which time the animals were killed. Lymphomas occurred in 8/33 males, an
incidence significantly different from that in controls (P<0.001). No
increase in tumour incidence was reported in females (Weisburger *et al.*,
1975).

3.2 Other relevant biological data

The i.p. LD$_{50}$ for chlorambucil given as a suspension in 0.5% carboxymethylcellulose to adult female Wistar rats was 23 mg/kg bw (Chaube *et al.*,
1967). Hebborn *et al.* (1965) reported an i.p. LD$_{50}$ of 28 mg/kg bw (acute
dose) and an i.m. LD$_{50}$ of 5 daily injections of 10 mg/kg bw (subacute dose)
in adult Holzmann rats. Severe bone-marrow depletion was produced in rats
by i.p. injections of 15 mg/kg bw chlorambucil. I.v. administration to
dogs of 4 mg/kg bw caused severe leucopaenia, vomiting and diarrhoea by
the 7th day (Boyland *et al.*, 1961).

Application of chlorambucil to the skin of mice caused slight patchy
epidermal hyperplasia (Salaman & Roe, 1956). Repeated i.p. doses given to
mice resulted in testicular atrophy and decreased spermatogenic activity
in 39 weeks (Shimkin *et al.*, 1966).

Following its i.p. injection into rats, the concentration of chlorambucil in blood serum was maximal in 15 minutes, and the highest concentrations were found in the liver, kidney and lungs 15-30 minutes after injection. The drug was detectable up to 8-10 hours after its administration
(Telicenas *et al.*, 1971).

When 8 mg/kg bw ^{3}H-chlorambucil were administered subcutaneously to
Yoshida ascites sarcoma-bearing rats, the highest tritium concentration
after 1 hour was found in the liver; that in the kidneys was 63% of the
liver value. After 6 hours the level of radioactivity in the liver had
fallen by 52%, but in the kidneys it had increased by 25%. In the blood,

radioactivity was associated mainly with the plasma, which had maximum labelling at 6 hours. After 24 hours 60% of the administered activity was excreted in the urine, and less than 0.2% was found in the faeces (Hill & Riches, 1971).

Chlorambucil binds covalently to proteins, mainly through carboxyl groups, both *in vivo* and *in vitro* (Linford, 1962; Stacey *et al.*, 1958). Alkylation of DNA also occurs *in vitro* (Stacey *et al.*, 1958). Incorporation of radioactivity into the DNA and RNA of sensitive and resistant Yoshida ascites cells was maximal 12 hours after s.c. injection of ^{3}H-chlorambucil in rats (Hill & Riches, 1971).

This chemical was teratogenic when administered intraperitoneally to rats on the 12th day of pregnancy in doses of 6, 8, 10 or 12 mg/kg bw. Abnormalities included exencephaly, cleft palate and deformed appendages, paws and tails. Histological examination showed injury to the nervous system, mesenchyma and liver (Chaube *et al.*, 1967; Murphy *et al.*, 1958).

Chlorambucil induces point mutations in *Escherichia coli* Sd-4-73 (Szybalski, 1958), mitotic gene conversion in the diploid strain D4 of *Saccharomyces cerevisiae* (Zimmermann, 1971) and chromosome aberrations of the chromatid type in short-term cultures of human peripheral lymphocytes (Reeves & Margoles, 1974).

Jaundice was observed in 3/29 patients treated with chlorambucil (Robert *et al.*, 1968).

A woman who became pregnant while receiving chlorambucil treatment (6 mg/day) had the pregnancy terminated at 3½ months; the left kidney and ureter were found to be absent in the foetus (Shotton *et al.*, 1963). Two other women treated with chlorambucil during pregnancy (in one case, 10 mg/day for 2 weeks at 4½ months and 10 mg/day for 4 weeks at 5-6 months; in the other case, 378 mg in 22 days at the 7th month) produced completely normal infants (Sokal & Lessmann, 1960).

3.3 Observations in man

A case of myelomonocytic leukaemia was reported in a patient who had received 4-5 mg/day chlorambucil for 40 months for the treatment of chronic

lymphocytic leukaemia (Catovsky & Galton, 1971). Two similar cases of
acute leukaemia occurred in patients with chronic lymphocytic leukaemia
who had been treated with chlorambucil for 2 and 3 years; in addition,
one patient had received numerous diagnostic X-rays and other radiation
therapy (McPhedran & Heath, 1970). Individual cases of acute myeloblastic
leukaemia (Tulliez *et al.*, 1974), erythroleukaemia (Laroche *et al.*, 1972),
reticulum-cell sarcoma (Österberg & Rausing, 1970), lymphosarcoma (Zittoun
et al., 1972) and transitional-cell carcinoma of the bladder (Dale & Smith,
1974) have been reported in patients with diseases other than cancer sub-
mitted to treatments including chlorambucil.

4.   Comments on Data Reported and Evaluation

4.1 Animal data

Chlorambucil is carcinogenic in mice and rats following its intraperitoneal injection, producing lymphomas in rats and lymphosarcomas,
ovarian tumours and a dose-related increase in the incidence of lung tumours
in mice.

4.2 Human data

The available case reports in which leukaemia and other tumours were
reported to have occurred in patients treated with chlorambucil provide
insufficient evidence to determine if there is an increased incidence of
cancer following the therapeutic use of this drug.

5. References

Baum, J. & Vaughan, J. (1969) Immunosuppressive drugs in rheumatoid arthritis. Ann. intern. Med., 71, 202-204

Boyland, E., Staunton, M.D. & Williams, K. (1961) Experimental regional administration (perfusion and infusion) of chlorambucil [p-N,N-di(β-chloroethyl)aminophenylbutyric acid]. Brit. J. Cancer, 15, 498-510

British Pharmaceutical Codex (1973) London, The Pharmaceutical Press

British Pharmacopoeia Commission (1973) British Pharmacopoeia, London, HMSO, pp. 93-94

Bundesverband der pharmazeutischen Industrie (1969) Rote Liste, Aulendorf/ Württ., Editio Cantor, p. 698

Catovsky, D. & Galton, D.A.G. (1971) Myelomonocytic leukaemia supervening on chronic lymphocytic leukaemia. Lancet, i, 478-479

Chaube, S., Kury, G. & Murphy, M.L. (1967) Teratogenic effects of cyclophosphamide (NSC-26271) in the rat. Cancer Chemother. Rep., 51, 363-376

Chemical Information Services, Ltd (1975) Directory of Western European Chemical Producers, 1975/76, Oceanside, NY

Dale, A.G. & Smith, R.B. (1974) Transitional cell carcinoma of the bladder associated with cyclophosphamide. J. Urol., 112, 603-604

Dictionnaire Vidal (1975) 51st ed., Paris, Office de Vulgarisation Pharmaceutique. p. 343

Everett, J.L., Roberts, J.R. & Ross, W.C.J. (1953) Aryl-2-halogenoalkylamines. XII. Some carboxylic derivatives of N,N-di-2-chloroethylaniline. J. chem. Soc. (Lond.), 2386-2392

Hebborn, P., Mishra, L.C., Dalton, C. & Williams, J.P.G. (1965) Dental lesions in rat induced by radiomimetic agents. Arch. Path., 80, 110-115

Hill, B.T. & Riches, P.G. (1971) The absorption, distribution and excretion of (^{3}H)-chlorambucil in rats bearing the Yoshida ascites sarcoma. Brit. J. Cancer, 25, 831-837

Huff, B.B., ed. (1974) Physicians' Desk Reference, 28th ed., Oradell, N.J., Medical Economics Co., p. 653

Kastrup, E.K., ed. (1974) Facts and Comparisons, St Louis, Missouri, Facts & Comparisons Inc., p. 386

Kozlov, N.E. & Bernshtein, V.N. (1968) Qualitative and quantitative analysis of drugs of the bis(2-chloroethyl)amine group. Aktual. Vop. Farm., 61-65

Laroche, Cl., Caquet, R. & Remy, J.-M. (1972) Erythroleucémie aiguë après traitement d'une exophtalmine maligne par le chlorambucil. Nouv. Presse méd., 1, 3133

Linford, J.H. (1961) Some interactions of nitrogen mustards with constituents of human blood serum. Biochem. Pharmacol., 8, 343-357

Linford, J.H. (1962) The recovery of free chlorambucil from solution in blood serum. Biochem. Pharmacol., 11, 693-706

McPhedran, P. & Heath, C.W., Jr (1970) Acute leukemia occurring during chronic lymphocytic leukemia. Blood, 35, 7-11

Murphy, M.L., Del Moro, A. & Lacon, C. (1958) The comparative effects of five polyfunctional alkylating agents on the rat fetus, with additional notes on the chick embryo. Ann. N.Y. Acad. Sci., 68, 762-782

Österberg, G. & Rausing, A. (1970) Reticulum cell sarcoma in Waldenström's macroglobulinemia after chlorambucil treatment. Acta med. scand., 188, 497-504

Phlippen, R., Schumacher, K., Gross, R. & Eder, M. (1969) Comparative studies on conventional and immunosuppressive therapy of chronic hepatitis treated with chlorambucil. Klin. Wschr., 47, 524-532

Pullom, E.N., ed. (1968-69) Mims Annual Compendium, London, Medical Publications Ltd, pp. 94-95

Reeves, B.R. & Margoles, C. (1974) Preferential location of chlorambucil-induced breakage in the chromosomes of normal human lymphocytes. Mutation Res., 26, 205-208

Robert, J., Barbier, P., Manaster, J. & Jacobs, E. (1968) Hepatotoxicity of cytostatic drugs evaluated by liver-function tests and appearance of jaundice. Digestion, 1, 229-232

Salaman, M.H. & Roe, F.J.C. (1956) Further tests for tumour-initiating activity: N,N-Di-(2-chloroethyl)-p-aminophenylbutyric acid (CB 1348) as an initiator of skin tumour formation in the mouse. Brit. J. Cancer, 10, 363-377

Shimkin, M.B., Weisburger, J.H., Weisburger, E.K., Gubareff, N. & Suntzeff, V. (1966) Bioassay of 29 alkylating chemicals by the pulmonary-tumor response in strain A mice. J. nat. Cancer Inst., 36, 915-935

Shotton, D., Lynchburg, V. & Monie, I.W. (1963) Possible teratogenic effect of chlorambucil on a human fetus. J. Amer. med. Ass., 186, 74-75

Sokal, J.E. & Lessmann, E.M. (1960) Effects of cancer chemotherapeutic agents on the human fetus. J. Amer. med. Ass., 172, 1765-1771

Stacey, K.A., Cobb, M., Cousens, S.F. & Alexander, P. (1958) The reactions of the "radiomimetic" alkylating agents with macromolecules *in vitro*. Ann. N.Y. Acad. Sci., 68, 682-701

Stecher, P.G., ed. (1968) The Merck Index, 8th ed., Rahway, N.J., Merck & Co., p. 232

Steinböck, R., Zekert, F. & Zimmermann, G. (1969) Austria-Codex: 1969/70, Vienna, Österreichischer Apotheker-Verlag, p. 441

Szybalski, W. (1958) Special microbiological systems. II. Observations on chemical mutagenesis in microorganisms. Ann. N.Y. Acad. Sci., 76, 475-489

Telicenas, A., Zebenkiene, B., Didzepetriene, J., Suminas, M. & Paulaitite, N. (1971) Distribution of lophenal, chlorambucil and hisphene. Kova, Veziu Tarybu Lietuvoje , 154-155

Tulliez, M., Ricard, M.F., Jan, F. & Sultan, C. (1974) Preleukaemic abnormal myelopoiesis induced by chlorambucil. A case study. Scand. J. Haemat., 13, 179-183

US Pharmacopeial Convention, Inc. (1970) The US Pharmacopeia, 18th rev., Easton, Pa., Mack

Weisburger, J.H., Griswold, D.P., Jr, Prejean, J.D., Casey, A.E., Wood, H.B., Jr & Weisburger, E.K. (1975) The carcinogenic properties of some of the principal drugs used in clinical cancer chemotherapy. Recent Results Cancer Res. (in press)

Zimmermann, F.K. (1971) Induction of mitotic gene conversion by mutagens. Mutation Res., 11, 327-337

Zittoun, R., Debri, P., Gardais, J., Thuan, F.P., Renier, J.C. & Simon, F. (1972) Lymphosarcome du grêle après traitement d'une polyarthrite rhumatoïde par le chlorambucil. Nouv. Presse méd., 1, 2477-2479

CYCLOPHOSPHAMIDE

1. Chemical and Physical Data

1.1 Synonyms and trade names

Chem. Abstr. Reg. Serial No.: 50-18-0

Chem. Abstr. Name: N,N-Bis(2-chloroethyl)tetrahydro-2H-1,3,2-oxa-phosphorin-2-amine, 2-oxide monohydrate

B 518; 1-bis(2-chloroethyl)amino-1-oxo-2-aza-5-oxaphosphoridine monohydrate; 2-[bis(2-chloroethyl)amino]-1-oxa-3-aza-2-phosphocyclo-hexane 2-oxide monohydrate; 2-[bis(2-chloroethyl)amino]tetrahydro-[2H]-1,3,2-oxazaphosphorine 2-oxide monohydrate; [bis(chloro-2-ethyl)-amino]-2-tetrahydro-3,4,5,6-oxazaphosphorine-1,3,2-oxide-2 monohydrate; N,N-bis(2-chloroethyl)-N'-(3-hydroxypropyl)phosphorodiamidic acid intramolecular ester monohydrate; bis(2-chloroethyl)phosphoramide cyclic propanolamide ester monohydrate; N,N-bis(β-chloroethyl)-N',O-propylenephosphoric acid ester amide monohydrate; N,N-bis(β-chloro-ethyl)-N',O-trimethylenephosphoric acid ester diamide monohydrate; CB-4564; cyclic N',O-propylene ester of N,N-bis(2-chloroethyl)phos-phorodiamidic acid monohydrate; cyclophosphamid; 2-[di(2-chloroethyl) amino]-1-oxa-3-aza-2-phosphacyclohexane-2-oxide monohydrate; N,N-di(2-chloroethyl)amino-N,O-propylene phosphoric acid ester diamide monohydrate; NSC-26271

B 518; Clafen; Cyclophosphamidum; Cyclophosphan; Cyclophosphane; Cyclophosphanum; Cytophosphan; Cytoxan; Endoxan; Endoxana; Endoxan-Asta; Endoxan R; Enduxan; Genoxal; Mitoxan; Procytox; Semdoxan; Sendoxan; Senduxan

1.2 Chemical formula and molecular weight

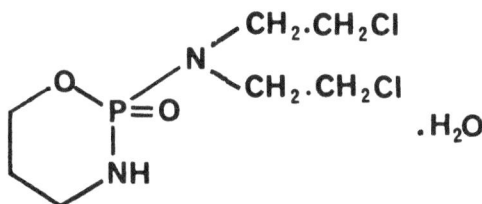

$C_7H_{15}Cl_2N_2O_2P \cdot H_2O$

Mol. wt: 279.1

1.3 Chemical and physical properties of the pure substance

(a) Description: A fine, white, odourless or almost odourless, crystalline powder with a slightly bitter taste. If the water of crystallization is removed by high vacuum or drying agents, it becomes an oily, half-liquid mass.

(b) Melting-point: 49.5-53°C, determined on the substance without previous drying (British Pharmacopoeia Commission, 1973)

(c) Spectroscopy data: IR spectrum (cm^{-1}) 3385 (N-H) (in dichloro-ethane) (Rauen, 1964)

(d) Solubility: Soluble at 20°C in 25 parts of water and in 1 part of ethanol; also soluble in benzene, chloroform, dioxane and glycols; slightly soluble in ether and acetone; insoluble in carbon tetrachloride and carbon disulphide (British Pharmacopoeia Commission, 1973; White, 1959)

(e) Stability: Darkens on exposure to light. Aqueous solutions may be kept for a few hours at room temperature, but hydrolysis occurs at temperatures above 30°C, with removal of chlorine atoms (British Pharmaceutical Codex, 1973).

1.4 Technical products and impurities

Cyclophosphamide is available in the US as a USP grade in the form of tablets containing 25 and 50 mg active ingredient, and in a crystalline hydrate form for injection packaged in ampoules in strengths of 100, 200 and 500 mg to be administered after solution in sterile water (Medical Economics Co., 1974). Cyclophosphamide crystalline hydrate USP, used to formulate the tablets and injections, contains 100±5% cyclophosphamide. The tablets contain 100±10% of the labelled amount of cyclophosphamide, and the injection, a sterile mixture with sodium chloride, contains 100±5% of the labelled amount of cyclophosphamide (US Pharmacopeial Convention, Inc., 1970).

In Europe, cyclophosphamide tablets are available in 10 and 50 mg strengths. The crystalline hydrate form for injection is available in ampoules containing 100, 200, 500 and 1000 mg active ingredient, to be

136

administered after solution in sterile water (Bundesverband der pharmazeutischen Industrie, 1969; *Dictionnaire Vidal*, 1975; Pullom, 1968-69).

In Japan, tablets containing 50 mg and ampoules for injection in 100,
200 and 500 mg strengths are available (JAPTA, 1973).

2. Production, Use, Occurrence and Analysis

For important background information on this section, see preamble,
p. 17.

2.1 Production and use

Cyclophosphamide can be prepared by treating N,N-bis(β-chloroethyl)-
phosphamide dichloride with propanolamine in the presence of trimethylamine
and dioxane (Arnold & Bourseaux, 1958).

The major producer of cyclophosphamide is in the Federal Republic of
Germany. Some of the production is exported to the US, where one company
has formulated and marketed the drug since 1959. Total US sales are
approximately 600 kg annually. Cyclophosphamide is also produced in
Finland and in the UK (Chemical Information Services, Ltd, 1975) where
production was estimated to have reached a few hundred kg annually in the
early seventies. Cyclophosphamide is also marketed in Japan.

Cyclophosphamide is the most widely used antineoplastic agent in the
treatment of various neoplastic diseases, including malignant lymphomas,
multiple myeloma, leukaemias, mycosis fungoides, neuroblastoma, adenocarcinoma of the ovary, retinoblastoma, carcinoma of the breast and malignant
neoplasms of the lung. It has been used in combination with other agents
to treat lymphoreticular and some other tumours (Greenwald, 1973;
Livingston & Carter, 1970). The usual initial dose is about 10 mg/kg bw
daily given intravenously for 2-5 days or 1-5 mg/kg bw daily given orally
(Medical Economics Co., 1974).

Cyclophosphamide is used in human medicine as an immunosuppressive
agent in a variety of non-malignant diseases, e.g., rheumatoid arthritis,
systemic lupus erythematosus, Wegener's granulomatosis, polymyositis, sclero-
derma, uveitis, idiopathic pulmonary hemosiderosis, glomerulonephritis,

idiopathic nephrotic syndrome in children, chronic interstitial pneumonia, psoriatic arthritis, Behcet's disease, pyoderma gangrenosum, myasthenia gravis, multiple sclerosis, idiopathic thrombocytopenic purpura, macroglobulinaemia and cryoglobulinaemia in Sjögren's syndrome, pemphigus vulgaris and bullous pemphigoid (Essig *et al.*, 1974; Medved & Maxwell, 1974; O'Donohue, 1974; Rubens-Duval *et al.*, 1974; Steinberg *et al.*, 1972). Recently, patients suffering from chronic hepatitis have also been treated with cyclophosphamide for long periods of time (Naccarato *et al.*, 1974). It is increasingly being used as an immunosuppressive agent following organ transplantation (Starzl *et al.*, 1973).

Cooperative trials with many hundreds of patients have been conducted to test its applicability in rheumatoid arthritis, nephrotic syndrome in children and systemic lupus erythematosus (Anon., 1974; Cooperating Clinics Committee, 1970; Mackay *et al.*, 1974).

Cyclophosphamide has also been tested as an insect chemosterilant (LaBrecque & Gouck, 1963). The US Department of Agriculture has shown it to be an effective agent for the removal of wool in the chemical shearing of sheep, and at the time of preparation of this monograph, application had been made to the US Food and Drug Administration for approval of its use in this way.

2.2 Occurrence

Cyclophosphamide is not known to occur in nature.

2.3 Analysis

Methods for the determination of cyclophosphamide include: one based on estimation of nitrogen, phosphorous or chloride content; colorimetric analysis, based on the intensity of a cobalt thiocyanate-cyclophosphamide complex or by use of 4-(4'-nitrobenzyl)pyridine after hydrolysis; titrimetric analysis, after precipitation of the digested material by quinoline and citric-molybdic acid solution; and infrared spectrometry. The method with the greatest degree of specificity is infrared spectrometry based on the characteristic stretching frequency of the phosphorous-oxygen bond at 9.5 μm (Boughton *et al.*, 1972).

A gas-liquid chromatographic determination of cyclophosphamide in raw material, tablets and drug-containing vials ready for injection has been reported by Boughton *et al.* (1972). Under the conditions specified by the authors, a chromatogram with three peaks is found: the two major peaks were identified by mass spectrometry as intact cyclophosphamide (the 90% peak, with a molecular ion of 260 mass units) and as dehydrohalogenated cyclophosphamide (the 9% peak, with a molecular ion of 224 mass units). Duncan *et al.* (1973) described a mass spectrometric method for studying the distribution of cyclophosphamide in human tissue and body fluids. A concentration of at least 1 μg/ml of body fluid was required in order to obtain a low-resolution spectrum in which the drug could be recognized: the spectrum is characterized by a weak molecular ion peak at m/e 260, with the most abundant fragment ion occurring at m/e 211, corresponding to loss of the $.CH_2Cl$ radical.

3. Biological Data Relevant to the Evaluation of Carcinogenic Risk to Man

3.1 Carcinogenicity and related studies in animals

(a) Subcutaneous and/or intramuscular administration

Mouse: Two groups of 10 male and 10 female 4-24-week old NZB/NZW hybrid mice, which develop autoimmune complex nephritis, were given daily s.c. injections of 1 mg/kg bw or 8 mg/kg bw cyclophosphamide in saline for up to 93 weeks; 20 males and 20 females were injected with saline alone and served as controls. Fifty percent of female controls had died by the 31st week of the study, compared with 41 and 60 weeks for those given the low and high dose levels. Fifty percent of male controls had died by 57 weeks, compared with 71 and 80 weeks for the treated animals. Tumours were observed in treated males after 60 weeks of treatment and in females after 40 weeks. Eight males and 9 females given the highest dose level developed lymphoreticular neoplasms together with local tumours, including squamous-cell carcinomas of the skin, lymphomas, a rhabdomyosarcoma and unclassified cutaneous tumours. Pulmonary adenomas were also observed in 4 mice. Of mice given the low dose level, 3 males and 2 females developed tumours, as did 2 male and 1 female controls (Walker & Bole, 1973a,b).

In a similar experiment, 6/10 high-dose treated females developed neoplasms, mainly lymphoreticular, after 36-64 weeks of treatment, compared with 0/16 controls. The average lifespans were 67 weeks in treated animals and 48 weeks in controls (Walker & Bole, 1971).

A group of 50 female NMRI mice, 65 days old, received 52 weekly s.c. injections of 26 mg/kg bw (7% of LD_{50}) cyclophosphamide (total dose, 1352 mg/kg bw); the average lifespan of treated animals was 630±130 days. In a control group, 3/46 (6%) mice developed stem-cell leukaemia; no other malignant tumours were observed. Of the treated mice, 28/46 (61%) developed tumours: 3 leukaemias, 12 mammary carcinomas and 1 other mammary tumour, 4 ovarian carcinomas, 1 fibrosarcoma of the thorax, 1 skin carcinoma, 2 carcinomas at the injection site and 4 lung tumours (Schmähl & Osswald, 1970). [P<0.001].

(b) Intraperitoneal administration

Mouse: Four groups of 15 male and 15 female A/J mice, 4-6 weeks of age, were given i.p. injections of cyclophosphamide in water 3 times per week for 4 weeks (total doses, 449, 144, 36 and 9 mg/kg bw). Of 385 male and 392 female controls receiving vehicle, 39.5% male and 31.4% female survivors developed lung tumours within 39 weeks, the numbers of tumours per mouse being 0.5 and 0.36. Survivors among treated animals after 39 weeks were 4/30, 27/30, 26/30 and 30/30, at the respective dose levels. The numbers of mice with lung tumours were 2 (50%; 2.5 tumours/mouse), 20 (74%; 1.3 tumours/mouse), 11 (42%; 0.6 tumours/mouse) and 12 (40%; 0.4 tumours/mouse), respectively. In the same experiment, cyclophosphamide was reported to be about 380 times less potent than uracil mustard on a molar basis (Shimkin *et al.*, 1966). [The incidence of lung tumours in treated mice was significantly greater than that in controls only for those given the second highest dose level (P<0.001).]

A group of 29 dd mice and a group of 25 A mice of both sexes, 4-5 weeks old, received i.p. injections of 5 mg/kg bw cyclophosphamide in saline twice weekly for 15 successive weeks; 20 and 16 control mice of each strain were injected with isotonic saline. All mice were observed until natural death. Tumours developed in various organs in 12/22 dd mice surviving more than 48 weeks after the beginning of the treatment; 3/10 control mice surviving beyond the same period also had tumours. Tumours developed in 6/16 A mice surviving more than 42 weeks, and in 2/11 control mice. In dd mice, the induced tumours were mainly in the lung, liver, testis and mammary gland; in A mice the tumours were in the lungs ($P>0.05$) (Tokuoka, 1965).

Two groups of 25 male and 25 female Swiss mice, 6 weeks old, were given thrice weekly i.p. injections of 12 or 25 mg/kg bw for 6 months and were observed for a further 12 months, at which time the animals were killed. Lung tumours occurred in 7/30 males and in 10/35 females, and bladder papillomas were found in 4/30 males. The incidences of each tumour type were statistically greater than those in controls ($P<0.05$) (Weisburger *et al.*, 1975).

Rat: Two groups of 25 male and 25-28 female Charles River CD rats were given thrice weekly i.p. injections of 5 or 10 mg/kg bw for 6 months and were observed for a further 12 months, at which time the animals were killed. Mammary carcinomas occurred in 9/53 females and in 1/50 males, and mammary adenomas occurred in 24/53 females. The results were statistically significant in treated females as compared with controls ($P<0.035$) (Weisburger *et al.*, 1975).

Newborn or preweanling mouse: The carcinogenicity of cyclophosphamide was compared with that of urethane by i.p. administration of isotonic saline, 0.8, 4.0 or 20.0 mg/kg bw cyclophosphamide or 700 mg/kg bw urethane to groups of 30 male and 30 female Charles River CD-1 mice within 24 hours of birth and again at 3 and 6 days of age. Mice which died during the study or were sacrificed at 79 weeks were examined grossly and microscopically. Urethane was found to be highly carcinogenic, but cyclophosphamide was neither leukaemogenic nor hepatocarcinogenic. The incidence of pulmonary adenomas was slightly but significantly greater than that in controls in males treated with the medium dose of cyclophosphamide (4/27 *versus* 0/28; $P<0.05$) (Kelly *et al.*, 1974).

(c) Intravenous administration

Rat: Schmähl (1967) reported an increased incidence of benign and malignant neoplasms in BR46 male rats, 3 months old, given 15 mg/kg bw (7% of the LD$_{50}$) cyclophosphamide intravenously once weekly for 50 weeks and observed until death. The 40 treated animals received a total dose of 750 mg/kg bw cyclophosphamide, and the average observation time of tumours was 18 months. Tumours (9 malignant and 5 benign) occurred in 54% (14/26) of treated animals and in 2% (1/50) of control animals (1 benign) [P<0.001]. In two further experiments, 65 control male rats had incidences of 5% (3/65) benign and 6% (4/65) malignant tumours; and 36 male rats given 52 weekly i.v. injections of 13 mg/kg bw cyclophosphamide had incidences of 11% (4/36) benign and 17% (6/36) malignant tumours [P>0.05]. Male rats given 5 doses of 33 mg/kg bw every two weeks had incidences of benign and malignant tumours of 8% (5/66) and 24% (16/66), respectively [P<0.01]. The average observation time of the tumours in treated rats was 16-18 months, and that in controls, 23 months (Schmähl & Osswald, 1970).

A group of 32 male Sprague-Dawley rats, 3 months old, received weekly i.v. injections of 13 mg/kg bw cyclophosphamide (total dose, 670 mg/kg bw). A group of 52 untreated rats served as controls. Malignant tumours developed in 14/32 treated rats within 510±90 days: there were 3 reticulum-cell sarcomas, 6 haemangioendotheliomas in various organs, 1 neurogenic sarcoma of the mediastinum, 1 sarcoma of the heart and 1 leukaemia; two rats had 2 malignant tumours each: one had an osteosarcoma of the paranasal sinus and a pheochromocytoma, and the other had an angiosarcoma of the abdomen and a pheochromocytoma. Of the controls, 6/52 developed malignant tumours within 670±150 days: 3 reticulum-cell sarcomas, 1 pheochromocytoma, 1 haemangiosarcoma of the lung and 1 sarcoma of the kidney (Schmähl, 1974). [P<0.001].

(d)   Other experimental systems

Pre- and postnatal exposure: A group of female mice consisting of two inbred strains was given i.p. doses of 25 mg/kg bw cyclophosphamide every 2 weeks over 60 weeks; the maximum survival was 2 years (total dose, 750 mg). Five hepatomas, 12 lung carcinomas and 1 skin carcinoma occurred among 33 mice surviving after 60 weeks. During the experiment these females were allowed to breed, and the offspring were either treated with 25 mg/kg bw cyclophosphamide every 14 days (total dose, 750 mg/kg bw) or left untreated.

142

Of treated males 16 mice survived 60 weeks or more; 2 developed lung adenomas and 3, lung carcinomas. Of treated females 18 survived 60 weeks or more; 1 developed a lung adenoma, 4, lung carcinomas, 3, hepatomas, 1, a skin carcinoma and 1, a skin sarcoma. In untreated offspring, lung adenomas occurred in 4/16 males and in 5/12 females surviving up to 18 months; 1 male and 2 females developed hepatomas; no lung carcinomas were observed. The incidences of lung adenomas and carcinomas in untreated female and male mice of these two strains were reported to be about 9% and 5% (Roschlau & Justus, 1971). [No statistical evaluation was possible.]

3.2 Other relevant biological data

The single i.v. LD_{50} has been reported to be 160 mg/kg bw for rats, 400 mg/kg bw for guinea-pigs, 130 mg/kg bw for rabbits and 40 mg/kg bw for dogs. The single oral LD_{50} is 180 mg/kg bw for rats (Brock & Wilmanns, 1958).

In mice, rats and dogs the predominant haematologic effect was leuco-paenia; some depression of the bone marrow and thrombocytes was also noted (Wheeler et al., 1962). A single i.p. dose of cyclophosphamide causes a marked necrosis of the bladder and of the tubular and pelvic epithelium in mice, rats and dogs (Campobasso & Berrino, 1972; Koss, 1967; Philips et al., 1961); relatively little damage was observed in liver (Lavin & Koss, 1971), even after prolonged administration (Hegewald & Bärenwald, 1972).

Necrosis of bladder tissue is followed by a rapid epithelial regeneration of diploid cells and later by the production of tetraploid, octoploid and occasional hyperploid cells (Clayson & Cooper, 1969; Locher & Cooper, 1970). Cyclophosphamide induced abnormal mitoses when it was administered to rats immediately after partial hepatectomy (Mietkiewski et al., 1973). In rats the drug is rapidly absorbed from blood, and the specific activity in various tissues is highest within the first 20-30 minutes following its injection. Up to 75% of injected radioactivity is excreted in the urine within 5-8 hours, and the compound is rapidly metabolized (Chandramouli & Sivaramakrishnan, 1969; Graul et al., 1967; Mosienko & Pivnyuk, 1968). The pharmacological properties of cyclophosphamide differ in neonatal and adult female Swiss-Webster mice: plasma radioactivity in neonatal mice is

143

highest 32 minutes after s.c. injection of the drug, and its half-life is 8.8 hours; in adults the half-life of plasma radioactivity is only 1.9 hours (Bus *et al.*, 1973).

Cyclophosphamide is not an alkylating agent as such, and it requires metabolic activation *in vitro* and *in vivo* (Brock & Hohorst, 1963). The predominant site of its activity is the liver, and its activation depends on the hepatic microsomal mixed-function oxidase system, requiring NADPH and oxygen (Brock & Hohorst, 1963; Cohen & Jao, 1970; Foley *et al.*, 1961; Sladek, 1971). Similar reactions may occur in bone marrow, kidney and tumour tissues (Kondo & Muragishi, 1970).

Other drugs, such as barbiturates or corticosteroids, have been found to affect cyclophosphamide metabolism and may consequently alter its toxicity and cytostatic activity (Hart & Adamson, 1969; Sladek, 1972).

Intermediates of cyclophosphamide formed by the mixed-function oxidase system include aldophosphamide, which tautomerizes to 4-hydroxycyclophosphamide and is further converted by a soluble liver enzyme to carboxyphosphamide, the major urinary metabolite. Of all identified metabolites, including 4-ketocyclophosphamide, only aldophosphamide has alkylating and cytotoxic activity (Bakke *et al.*, 1972; Hill *et al.*, 1972; Hohorst *et al.*, 1971; Sladek, 1973; Struck *et al.*, 1971).

Alternatively, it has been suggested that cyclophosphamide is first converted into 4-hydroxycyclophosphamide, which may then break down by elimination of acrolein from its tautomeric form, aldophosphamide, to yield phosphoramide mustard. In competition with this process, the enzymic conversion of 4-hydroxycyclophosphamide to 4-ketocyclophosphamide by dehydrogenation and of aldophosphamide to carboxyphosphamide by oxidation may occur. On the basis of a bioassay involving Walker tumour cells in whole animals, Connors *et al.* (1974) have claimed that phosphoramide mustard possesses the cytotoxic properties of the active anti-tumour metabolite.

Reactive cyclophosphamide metabolites have been shown to cross-link nucleic acids; *in vitro* and *in vivo* studies indicate that the major reaction site is the 7-position of guanine (Campbell, 1968; Wheeler, 1962).

144

Cyclophosphamide is teratogenic in several species, including mice, rats, rabbits and chicks. It produces a variety of skeletal, soft tissue and other malformations and an increased number of resorptions; the type and frequency of malformations are strictly dose- and time-dependent (Gibson & Becker, 1968; Kreybig, 1965; Singh, 1971).

Placental transfer of ^{14}C-cyclophosphamide has been demonstrated in mice (Gibson & Becker, 1971), and a positive correlation between the alkylation of embryonic DNA and production of congenital abnormalities has been reported by Murthy et al. (1973). A similar correlation has been found for nuclear-DNA-dependent RNA polymerases in rat embryos (Köhler & Merker, 1973).

Reactive cyclophosphamide metabolites were bound to DNA, RNA and proteins isolated from embryos and livers of pregnant mice, and the extent of this binding was found to be modified by phenobarbital and by 2-diethyl-aminoethyl-2,2-diphenyl valerate (Murthy et al., 1973).

Cyclophosphamide induces point mutations in several genes of *Escherichia coli* 343/113 after activation by mouse and rat liver fractions (Ellenberger & Mohn, 1975). In a host-mediated assay using rats and mice, point mutations in bacteria (Propping et al., 1972) and mitotic gene conversions in strain D4 of *Saccharomyces cerevisiae* (Fahrig, 1974) were induced. Urinary metabolites from cyclophosphamide-treated rats induced mitotic gene conversions in *Saccharomyces cerevisiae* D4 (Siebert, 1974). Cyclophosphamide induces dominant lethal mutations in C3H mice (Röhrborn & Vogel, 1967) and recessive lethal mutations in Muller-5 strain of *Drosophila melanogaster* (Bertram & Höhne, 1959). Chromosome aberrations are induced in human peripheral white blood cells after cyclophosphamide treatment with a cumulative dose of about 10 g over a period of 6 weeks (Bauchinger & Schmid, 1969).

Cyclophosphamide can cause sterility in either sex in man. It can damage germinal cells in prepubertal and pubertal males (Penso et al., 1974) and accounts for premature ovarian failure in females (Uldall et al., 1972). The predominant haematologic effect of this drug is leucopaenia (Bergsagel et al., 1968). The reported incidence of cystitis in patients treated with cyclophosphamide ranges from 4-36% (Bennett, 1974).

145

The distribution of cyclophosphamide in the body and its metabolism appear to be similar in man and animals (Brock *et al.*, 1971). After its i.v. injection the drug is rapidly absorbed from the blood: in patients receiving 6-80 mg/kg bw/day of radio-labelled cyclophosphamide i.v., the radioactivity was distributed rapidly to all tissues: its half-life in the plasma was 6.5 hours; 68% of the injected label was excreted in the urine within 4 days; no radioactivity was found in the expired air or in the faeces (Bagley *et al.*, 1973). Ten to 14% of the drug is excreted unchanged (Bolt *et al.*, 1961; Cohen *et al.*, 1971); 56% of the reactive metabolites were bound to plasma proteins. Cyclophosphamide and several of its metabolites have also been found in bile, milk, sweat, saliva, cerebrospinal fluid and synovial fluid (Duncan *et al.*, 1973; Wiernik & Duncan, 1971). The metabolism of intravensouly administered ^{14}C-cyclophosphamide and the rate of excretion of its metabolites show large individual variations (Mouridsen *et al.*, 1974).

The drug is most toxic to the human foetus during the first 3 months, and congenital abnormalities have been detected after i.v. injection of large doses to pregnant women during this period of pregnancy (Greenberg & Tanaka, 1964; Toledo *et al.*, 1971).

3.3 Observations in man

At least 10 cases of malignant tumours have been reported in patients treated with cyclophosphamide for non-malignant disorders, and in 8 of these it was the only chemotherapeutic agent administered. The condition most commonly treated was the nephrotic syndrome, and the duration of cyclophosphamide therapy (when stated) was 3-24 months with an interval of 2 months to 3 or more years between the start of treatment and diagnosis of the tumour. The 8 tumours comprised 2 cases of reticulum-cell sarcoma (Fosdick *et al.*, 1969; Tannenbaum & Schur, 1974) and one case each of chronic lymphocytic leukaemia (Fosdick *et al.*, 1969), Hodgkin's disease (Cameron *et al.*, 1974), cervical cancer (Bashour *et al.*, 1973), malignant melanoma (Manny *et al.*, 1972), astrocytoma (Cameron *et al.*, 1974) and glioblastoma (Starzl *et al.*, 1973). In the two other cases a transitional-cell carcinoma of the bladder (Dale & Smith, 1974) and a reticulum-cell sarcoma (Worrledge *et al.*, 1968) developed after cyclophosphamide and chlorambucil

146

chemotherapy; in the latter case the patient was treated for autoimmune haemolytic anaemia, which may have been the first manifestation of the reticulum-cell sarcoma. In addition, there have been 16 reports of second primary tumours following cyclophosphamide therapy for the treatment of malignant diseases; in 6 cases cyclophosphamide was the only chemotherapy used, and in 5 cases irradiation was also administered (Dale & Smith, 1974; Greenspan & Tung, 1974; Karchmer *et al.*, 1974; Mundy & Baikie, 1973; Okano *et al.*, 1966; River & Schorr, 1966; Sypkens-Smit & Meyler, 1970; Worth, 1971). The duration of treatment with cyclophosphamide in these cases was from 1-48 months or more. The 6 second primary tumours which followed chemotherapy with cyclophosphamide alone were 3 carcinomas of the bladder (Dale & Smith, 1974; Worth, 1971), 2 cases of acute leukaemia, both in myeloma patients (Karchmer *et al.*, 1974), 1 reticulum-cell sarcoma (Mundy & Baikie, 1973). Two cases of plasma-cell reticulosarcoma involving non-lymphoreticular tissues were seen in patients with myeloma receiving cyclophosphamide therapy only (Holt & Robb-Smith, 1973)[1].

A current prospective study of patients with non-malignant disorders and who were treated with immunosuppressive drugs (Doll & Kinlen, 1970) has so far produced no evidence of an increased incidence of malignant disease in patients treated with cyclophosphamide (Cameron, 1975).

---

[1]Note by the Secretariat:

    Prior to publication of this volume an article appeared describing five further cases of bladder cancer in patients with myeloma or Hodgkin's disease who had been treated with cyclophosphamide only in four cases, and with cyclophosphamide plus chlorambucil in one case, for 3-6 years [Wall, R.L. & Clausen, K.P. (1975) Carcinoma of the urinary bladder in patients receiving cyclophosphamide. New Engl. J. Med., iii, 271-273].

4. Comments on Data Reported and Evaluation

4.1 Animal data

Cyclophosphamide is carcinogenic in mice and rats following its intraperitoneal injection, in rats following its intravenous injection and in mice following its subcutaneous injection, in doses similar to those used in clinical practice. It produced mainly lung and lymphoreticular tumours, and also tumours of the liver and reproductive organs, sarcomas and squamous-cell carcinomas of the skin.

4.2 Human data

The available case reports in which tumours were reported to have occurred in patients treated with cyclophosphamide provide insufficient evidence to determine if there is an increased risk of cancer following the therapeutic use of this drug, with the possible exception of cancer of the bladder.

5. References

Anon. (1974) Prospective controlled trial of cyclophosphamide therapy in children with the nephrotic syndrome. Report of the International Study of Kidney Disease in Children. Lancet, ii, 423-427

Arnold, H. & Bourseaux, F. (1958) Synthese und Abbau cytostatisch wirksamer cyclischer *N*-Phosphamidester des Bis-(ß-Chloräthyl)amins. Angew. Chem., 70, 539-544

Bagley, C.M., Jr, Bostick, F.W. & DeVita, V.T., Jr (1973) Clinical pharmacology of cyclophosphamide. Cancer Res., 33, 226-233

Bakke, J.E., Feil, V.J., Fjelstul, C.E. & Thacker, E.J. (1972) Metabolism of cyclophosphamide by sheep. J. agric. Fd Chem., 20, 384-388

Bashour, B.N., Mancer, K. & Rance, C.P. (1973) Malignant mixed Mullerian tumor of the cervix following cyclophosphamide therapy for nephrotic syndrome. J. Pediat., 82, 292-293

Bauchinger, M. & Schmid, E. (1969) Cytogenetische Veränderungen in weissen Blutzellen nach Cyclophosphamidtherapie. Z. Krebsforsch., 72, 77-87

Bennett, A.H. (1974) Cyclophosphamide and hemorrhagic cystitis. J. Urol., 111, 603-606

Bergsagel, D.E., Robertson, G.L. & Hasselback, R. (1968) Effect of cyclophosphamide on advanced lung cancer and the hematological toxicity of large, intermittent intravenous doses. Canad. med. Ass. J., 98, 532-538

Bertram, C. & Höhne, G. (1959) Über die radiomimetische Wirkung einiger Zytostatika im Mutationsversuch an *Drosophila*. Strahlentherapie, 43, 388-391

Bolt, W., Ritzl, F., Toussaint, R. & Nahrmann, H. (1961) Verteilung und Ausscheidung eines cytostatisch wirkenden, mit Tritium markierten *N*-Lost-Derivates beim krebskranken Menschen. Arzneimittel-Forsch., 11, 170-175

Boughton, O.D., Brown, R.D., Bryant, R., Burger, F.J. & Combs, C.M. (1972) Assay of cyclophosphamide. J. pharm. Sci., 61, 97-100

British Pharmaceutical Codex (1973) London, The Pharmaceutical Press

British Pharmacopoeia Commission (1973) British Pharmacopoeia, London, HMSO, pp. 315-316

Brock, N. & Hohorst, H.J. (1963) Über die Aktivierung von Cyclophosphamid *in vivo* und *in vitro*. Arzneimittel-Forsch., 13, 1021-1031

Brock, N. & Wilmanns, H. (1958) Wirkung eines zyklischen *N*-Lost-Phosphamid-esters auf experimentell erzeugte Tumoren der Ratte. Dtsch. med. Wschr., 83, 453-458

Brock, N., Gross, R., Hohorst, H.J., Klein, H.O. & Schneider, B. (1971) Activation of cyclophosphamide in man and animals. Cancer, 27, 1512-1529

Bundesverband der pharmazeutischen Industrie (1969) Rote Liste, Frankfurt, p. 412

Bus, J.S., Short, R.D. & Gibson, J.E. (1973) Effect of phenobarbital and SKF 525 A on the toxicity, elimination and metabolism of cyclophosphamide in newborn mice. J. Pharmacol. exp. Ther., 184, 749-756

Cameron, J.S. (1975) Problems with immunosuppressive agents in renal disease. J. clin. Path., 28 (in press)

Cameron, J.S., Chantler, C., Ogg, C.S. & White, R.H.R. (1974) Long-term stability of remission in nephrotic syndrome after treatment with cyclophosphamide. Brit. med. J., iv, 7-11

Campbell, P.N. (1968) Interaction of Drugs and Subcellular Components in Animal Cells, London, Churchill

Campobasso, O. & Berrino, F. (1972) Early effects of cyclophosphamide on mouse bladder epithelium. Path. Microbiol., 38, 144-149

Chandramouli, K. & Sivaramakrishnan, V.M. (1969) Radiation and radiomimetic agents. I. The distribution of P^{32}-labelled cyclophosphamide in albino rats and in humans. Indian J. Cancer, 6, 153-164

Chemical Information Services, Ltd (1975) Directory of Western European Chemical Producers, 1975/76, Oceanside, NY

Clayson, D.B. & Cooper, E.H. (1969) The immediate response of bladder epithelium to injury by chemical carcinogens. Brit. J. Urol., 41, 710-713

Cohen, J.L. & Jao, J.Y. (1970) Enzymatic basis of cyclophosphamide activation by hepatic microsomes of the rat. J. Pharmacol. exp. Ther., 174, 206-210

Cohen, J.L., Jao, J.Y. & Jusko, W.J. (1971) Pharmacokinetics of cyclophosphamide in man. Brit. J. Pharmacol., 43, 677-680

Connors, T.A., Cox, P.J., Farmer, P.B., Foster, A.B. & Jarman, M. (1974) Some studies of the active intermediates formed in the microsomal metabolism of cyclophosphamide and isophosphamide. Biochem. Pharmacol., 23, 115-129

Cooperating Clinics Committee of the American Rheumatism Association (1970) A controlled trial of cyclophosphamide in rheumatoid arthritis. New Engl. J. Med., 283, 883-889

Dale, G.A. & Smith, R.B. (1974) Transitional-cell carcinoma of the bladder associated with cyclophosphamide. J. Urol., 112, 603-604

Dictionnaire Vidal (1975) 51st ed., Paris, Office de Vulgarisation Pharmaceutique, p. 511

Doll, R. & Kinlen, L. (1970) Immunosurveillance and cancer: epidemiological evidence. Brit. med. J., iv, 420-422

Duncan, J.H., Colvin, O.M. & Fenselau, C. (1973) Mass spectrometric study of the distribution of cyclophosphamide in humans. Toxicol. appl. Pharmacol., 24, 317-323

Ellenberger, J. & Mohn, G. (1975) Mutagenic activity of cyclophosphamide, ifosfamide and trofosfamide in different genes of *Escherichia coli* and *Salmonella typhimurium* after biotransformation through extracts of rodent liver. Arch. Toxikol. (in press)

Essig, L.J., Timms, E.S., Hancock, D.E. & Sharp, G.C. (1974) Plasma-cell interstitial pneumonia and macroglobulinemia. A response to corticosteroid and cyclophosphamide therapy. Amer. J. Med., 56, 398-405

Fahrig, R. (1974) Development of host-mediated mutagenicity tests. I. Differential response of yeast cells injected into the testes of rats and the peritoneum of mice and rats to mutagens. Mutation Res., 26, 29-36

Foley, G.E., Friedman, O.M. & Drolet, B.P. (1961) Studies on the mechanism of action of cytoxan. Evidence of activation *in vivo* and *in vitro*. Cancer Res., 21, 57-63

Fosdick, W.M., Parsons, J.L. & Hill, D.F. (1969) Long-term cyclophosphamide therapy in rheumatoid arthritis - a progress report, six years' experience. Arthritis-Rheum., 12, 663

Gibson, J.E. & Becker, B.A. (1968) The teratogenicity of cyclophosphamide in mice. Cancer Res., 28, 475-480

Gibson, J.E. & Becker, B.A. (1971) Effect of phenobarbital and SKF 525 A on placental transfer of cyclophosphamide in mice. J. Pharmacol. exp. Ther., 177, 256-262

Graul, E.H., Schaumlöffel, E., Hundeshagen, H., Wilmanns, H. & Simon, G. (1967) Metabolism of radioactive cyclophosphamide. Cancer, 20, 896-899

Greenberg, L.H. & Tanaka, K.R. (1964) Congenital anomalies probably induced by cyclophosphamide. J. Amer. med. Ass., 188, 423-426

Greenspan, E.M. & Tung, B.G. (1974) Acute myeloblastic leukemia after cure of ovarian cancer. J. Amer. med. Ass., 230, 418-420

Greenwald, E.S. (1973) Cancer Chemotherapy, 2nd ed., Bern, Hans Huber, pp. 121-133

Hart, L.G. & Adamson, R.H. (1969) Effect of microsomal enzyme modifiers on toxicity and therapeutic activity of cyclophosphamide in mice. Arch. int. Pharmacodyn., 180, 391-401

Hegewald, G. & Bärenwald, G. (1972) Morphologische Veränderungen der Rattenleber durch längerdauernde Zyklophosphamidgaben. Acta hepato-gastroenterol., 19, 85-90

Hill, D.L., Laster, W.R., Jr & Struck, R.F. (1972) Enzymatic metabolism of cyclophosphamide and nicotine and production of a toxic cyclophosphamide metabolite. Cancer Res., 32, 658-665

Hohorst, H.J., Ziemann, A. & Brock, N. (1971) 4-Ketocyclophosphamide, a metabolite of cyclophosphamide. Arzneimittel-Forsch., 21, 1254-1257

Holt, J.M. & Robb-Smith, A.H.T. (1973) Multiple myeloma: development of plasma cell sarcoma during apparently successful chemotherapy. J. clin. Path., 26, 649-659

JAPTA (Japan Pharmaceutical Traders Association) (1973) Japanese Drug Directory, Tokyo, p. 240

Karchmer, R.K., Amare, M., Larsen, W.E., Mallouk, A.G. & Caldwell, G.G. (1974) Alkylating agents as leukemogens in multiple myeloma. Cancer, 33, 1103-1107

Kelly, W.A., Nelson, L.W., Hawkins, H.C. & Weikel, J.H., Jr (1974) An evaluation of the tumorigenicity of cyclophosphamide and urethan in newborn mice. Toxicol. appl. Pharmacol., 27, 629-640

Köhler, E. & Merker, H.J. (1973) Effect of cyclophosphamide pretreatment of pregnant animals on the activity of nuclear DNA-dependent RNA polymerases in different parts of rat embryos. Naunyn-Schmiedeberg's Arch. exp. Path. Pharmak., 277, 71-88

Kondo, T. & Muragishi, H. (1970) Mechanism of cyclophosphamide activation. Gann, 61, 145-151

Koss, L.G. (1967) A light and electron microscopic study of the effects of a single dose of cyclophosphamide on various organs in the rat. I. The urinary bladder. Lab. Invest., 16, 44-65

Kreybig, T., von (1965) Die teratogene Wirkung von Cyclophosphamid während der embryonalen Entwicklungsphase bei der Ratte. Naunyn-Schmiedeberg's Arch. exp. Path. Pharmak., 252, 173-195

LaBrecque, G.C. & Gouck, H.K. (1963) Compounds affecting fertility in adult houseflies. J. econ. Entomol., 56, 476

Lavin, P. & Koss, L.G. (1971) Effects of a single dose of cyclophosphamide on various organs in the rat. III. Electron microscopic study of the liver. Amer. J. Path., 62, 159-168

Livingston, R.B. & Carter, S.K. (1970) Single Agents in Cancer Chemotherapy, New York, Plenum Press, pp. 25-80

Locher, G.W. & Cooper, E.H. (1970) Repair of rat urinary bladder epithelium following injury by cyclophosphamide. Invest. Urol., 8, 116-123

Mackay, I.R., Mathews, J.D., Toth, T.B.H., Baker, H.W.G. & Walker, I. (1974) A sequential trial comparing cyclophosphamide and azathioprine as adjuncts in the treatment of systemic lupus erythematosus. Aust. N.Z. J. Med., 4, 154-161

Manny, N., Rosenman, E. & Benbassat, J. (1972) Hazard of immunosuppressive therapy. Brit. med. J., ii, 291

Medical Economics Co. (1974) Physicians' Desk Reference, 28th ed., Oradell, NJ, p. 975

Medved, A. & Maxwell, I. (1974) Intermittent cyclophosphamide in pemphigus vulgaris and bullous pemphigoid. Canad. med. Ass. J., 111, 245-250

Mietkiewski, K., Karon, H. & Warchol, J.B. (1973) The effect of cyclophosphamide (endoxan) on histoenzymatic reactions in the liver. II. Studies on liver regeneration during cyclophosphamide administration. Acta histochem., 45, 185-198

Mosienko, V.S. & Pivnyuk, V.M. (1968) Distribution of thio-TEPA and cyclophosphamide in rats and their renal excretion. Vrach. Delo, 8, 52-54

Mouridsen, H.T., Faber, O. & Skovsted, L. (1974) The biotransformation of cyclophosphamide in man: analysis of the variation in normal subjects. Acta pharmacol., 35, 98-106

Mundy, G.R. & Baikie, A.G. (1973) Myeloma treated with cyclophosphamide and terminating in reticulum-cell sarcoma. Med. J. Austr., 1, 1240-1241

Murthy, V.V., Becker, B.A. & Steel, W.J. (1973) Effects of dosage, phenobarbital and 2-diethylaminoethyl-2,2-diphenylvalerate on the binding of cyclophosphamide and/or its metabolites to the DNA, RNA and protein of the embryo and liver in pregnant mice. Cancer Res., 33, 664-670

Naccarato, R., Farini, R., Chiaramonte, M., Fagiolo, U. & Sturniolo, G.C. (1974) Treatment of active chronic hepatitis with cyclophosphamide. Postgrad. med. J., 50, 16-24

O'Donohue, W.J. (1974) Idiopathic pulmonary hemosiderosis with manifestations of multiple connective tissue and immune disorders. Treatment with cyclophosphamide. Amer. Rev. resp. Dis., 109, 473-479

Okano, H., Azar, H.A. & Osserman, E.F. (1966) Plasmacytic reticulum cell sarcoma. Case report with electron microscopic studies. Amer. J. clin. Path., 46, 546-555

Penso, J., Lippe, B., Ehrlich, R. & Smith, F.G., Jr (1974) Testicular function in prepubertal and pubertal male patients treated with cyclophosphamide for nephrotic syndrome. J. Pediat., 84, 831-836

Philips, F.S., Sternberg, S.S., Cronin, A.P. & Vidal, P.M. (1961) Cyclophosphamide and urinary bladder toxicity. Cancer Res., 21, 1577-1589

Propping, P., Röhrborn, G. & Buselmaier, W. (1972) Comparative investigations on the chemical induction of point mutations and dominant lethal mutations in mice. Mol. gen. Genet., 117, 197-209

Pullom, E.N., ed. (1968-69) Mims Annual Compendium, London, Medical Publications Ltd, p. 336

Rauen, H.M. (1964) Biochemisches Taschenbuch, Berlin, Springer-Verlag, p. 89

River, G.L. & Schorr, W.F. (1966) Malignant skin tumors in multiple myeloma. Arch. Derm., 93, 432-438

Röhrborn, G. & Vogel, F. (1967) Mutationen durch chemische Einwirkung bei Säuger und Mensch. II. Genetische Untersuchungen an der Maus. Dtsch. med. Wschr., 92, 2315-2321

Roschlau, G. & Justus, J. (1971) Kanzerogene Wirkung von Methotrexat und Cyclophosphamid im Tierexperiment. Dtsch. Gesundheitsw., 26, 219-222

Rubens-Duval, A., Kaplan, G. & Nobillot, A. (1974) Cryoglobuline, macroglobuline et syndrome de Gougerot-Sjögren traitement par le chlorambucil et la cyclophosphamide. Sem. Hôp. Paris, 50, 1665-1671

Schmähl, D. (1967) Karcinogene Wirkung von Cyclophosphamid und Triazichon bei Ratten. Dtsch. med. Wschr., 92, 1150-1152

Schmähl, D. (1974) Investigations on the influence of immunodepressive means on the chemical carcinogenesis in rats. Z. Krebsforsch., 81, 211-215

Schmähl, D. & Osswald, H. (1970) Experimentelle Untersuchungen über carcinogene Wirkungen von Krebs-Chemotherapeutica und Immunosuppressiva. Arzneimittel-Forsch., 20, 1461-1467

Shimkin, M.B., Weisburger, J.H., Weisburger, E.K., Gubareff, N. & Suntzeff, V. (1966) Bioassay of 29 alkylating chemicals by the pulmonary-tumor response in strain A mice. J. nat. Cancer Inst., 36, 915-935

Siebert, D. (1974) Comparison of the genetic activity of cyclophosphamide, ifosfamide and trofosfamide in host-mediated assays with the gene conversion system of yeast. Z. Krebsforsch., 81, 261-268

Singh, S. (1971) The teratogenicity of cyclophosphamide (endoxan-asta) in rats. Indian J. med. Res., 59, 1128-1135

Sladek, N.E. (1971) Metabolism of cyclophosphamide by rat hepatic microsomes. Cancer Res., 31, 901-908

Sladek, N.E. (1972) Therapeutic efficacy of cyclophosphamide as a function of inhibition of its metabolism. Cancer Res., 32, 1848-1854

Sladek, N.E. (1973) Bioassay and relative cytotoxic potency of cyclophosphamide metabolites generated *in vitro* and *in vivo*. Cancer Res., 33, 1150-1158

Starzl, T.E., Groth, C.G., Putnam, C.W., Corman, J., Halgrimson, C.G., Penn, I., Husberg, B., Gustafsson, A., Cascardo, S., Geis, P. & Iwatsuki, S. (1973) Cyclophosphamide for clinical renal and hepatic transplantation. Transplant. Proc., 5, 511-516

Steinberg, A.D., Plotz, P.H., Wolff, S.M., Wong, V.G., Agus, S.G. & Decker, J.L. (1972) Cytotoxic drugs in treatment of nonmalignant diseases. Ann. int. Med., 76, 619-642

Struck, R.F., Kirk, M.C., Mellett, L.B., Dareer, S.E. & Hill, D.L. (1971) Urinary metabolites of the antitumor agent cyclophosphamide. Mol. Pharmacol., 7, 519-529

Sypkens-Smit, C.G. & Meyler, L. (1970) Acute myeloid leukaemia after treatment with cytostatic agents. Lancet, ii, 671-672

Tannenbaum, H. & Schur, P.H. (1974) Development of reticulum cell sarcoma during cyclophosphamide therapy. Arthritis-Rheum., 17, 15-18

Tokuoka, S. (1965) Induction of tumor in mice with N,N-bis(2-chloroethyl)-N',O-propylenephosphoric acid ester diamide (cyclophosphamide). Gann, 56, 537-541

Toledo, T.M., Harper, R.C. & Moser, R.H. (1971) Fetal effects during cyclophosphamide and irradiation therapy. Ann. int. Med., 74, 87-91

Uldall, P.R., Kerr, D.N.S. & Tacchi, D. (1972) Sterility and cyclophosphamide. Lancet, i, 693-694

US Pharmacopeial Convention, Inc. (1970) The US Pharmacopeia, 18th rev., Easton, Pa , Mack, pp. 159-161

Walker, S.E. & Bole, G.G., Jr (1971) Augmented incidence of neoplasia in female New Zealand black/New Zealand white (NZB/NZW) mice treated with long-term cyclophosphamide. J. Lab. clin. Med., 78, 978-979

155

Walker, S.E. & Bole, G.G., Jr (1973a) Augmented incidence of neoplasia in NZB/NZW mice treated with long-term cyclophosphamide. J. Lab. clin. Med., 82, 619-633

Walker, S.E. & Bole, G.G., Jr (1973b) Suppressed autoantibody response and development of lymphomas in NZB/NZW mice treated with long-term cyclophosphamide. Arthritis-Rheum., 16, 137

Weisburger, J.H., Griswold, D.P., Jr, Prejean, J.D., Casey, A.E., Wood, H.B., Jr & Weisburger, E.K. (1975) The carcinogenic properties of some of the principal drugs used in cancer chemotherapy. Recent Results Cancer Res. (in press)

Wheeler, A.G., Dansby, D., Hawkins, H.C., Payne, H.G. & Weikel, J.H., Jr (1962) A toxicologic and hematologic evaluation of cyclophosphamide (cytoxan) in experimental animals. Toxicol. appl. Pharmacol., 4, 324-343

Wheeler, G.P. (1962) Studies related to the mechanisms of action of cytotoxic alkylating agents: a review. Cancer Res., 22, 651-687

White, F.R. (1959) Cytoxan. Cancer Chemother. Rep., 3, 21-25

Wiernik, P.H. & Duncan, J.H. (1971) Cyclophosphamide in human milk. Lancet, i, 912

Worrledge, S.M., Brain, M.C., Cooper, A.C., Hobbs, J.R. & Dacie, J.V. (1968) Immunosuppressive drugs in the treatment of autoimmune haemolytic anaemia. Proc. roy. Soc. Med., 61, 1312-1315

Worth, P.H.L. (1971) Cyclophosphamide and the bladder. Brit. med. J., ii, 182

MANNOMUSTINE (DIHYDROCHLORIDE)

1. Chemical and Physical Data

Mannomustine (free base)

1.1 Synonyms and trade names

Chem. Abstr. Reg. Serial No.: 576-68-1

Chem. Abstr. Name: 1,6-Bis(2-chloroethylamino)-1,6-dideoxy-D-mannitol

1,6-Bis(chloroethylamino)-1,6-bis-deoxy-D-mannitol; 1,6-bis(chloro-ethylamino)-1,6-dideoxy-D-mannite; 1,6-bis[(β-chloroethyl)amino]-1,6-dideoxy-D-mannitol; mannitol mustard*; mannitol nitrogen mustard*

1.2 Chemical formula and molecular weight

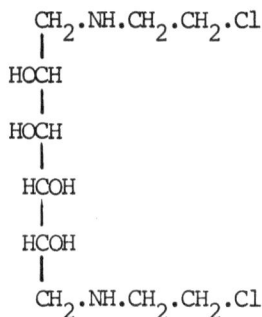

$$CH_2.NH.CH_2.CH_2.Cl$$
$$|$$
$$HOCH$$
$$|$$
$$HOCH$$
$$|$$
$$HCOH$$
$$|$$
$$HCOH$$
$$|$$
$$CH_2.NH.CH_2.CH_2.Cl$$

$C_{10}H_{22}Cl_2N_2O_4$ Mol. wt: 305

1.3 Chemical and physical properties of the pure substance

(a) Description: White crystals

(b) Melting-point: 278°C (decomposition)

(c) Solubility: Slightly soluble in water, ethanol and pyridine

1.4 Technical products and impurities

Mannomustine is not produced commercially.

---

*This name is also frequently used for the dihydrochloride salt of mannomustine.

Mannomustine dihydrochloride

1.1 Synonyms and trade names

Chem. Abstr. Reg. Serial No.: 551-74-6

Chem. Abstr. Name: 1,6-Bis(2-chloroethylamino)-1,6-dideoxy-D-mannitol dihydrochloride

BCM; 1,6-bis(chloroethylamino)-1,6-dideoxy-D-mannite; 1,6-bis(chloro-ethylamino)-1,6-dideoxy-D-mannite dihydrochloride; 1,6-bis(β-chloro-ethylamino)-1,6-dideoxy-D-mannitol dihydrochloride; 1,6-di(2-chloro-ethylamino)-1,6-dideoxy-D-mannitol dihydrochloride; 1,6-dideoxy-1,6-di(2-chloroethylamino)-D-mannitol dihydrochloride; dimesylmannitol; mannitol mustard*; mannitol nitrogen mustard*; mannogranol; mannomustine*; mannomustine hydrochloride; NSC 9698

Degranol; Degranol Chinoin

1.2 Chemical formula and molecular weight

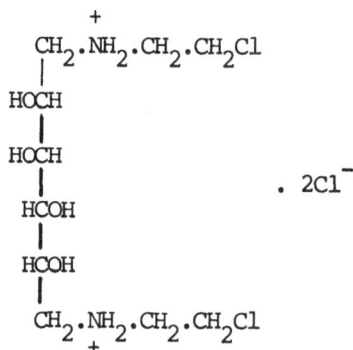

$$CH_2.\overset{+}{N}H_2.CH_2.CH_2Cl$$
$$|$$
$$HOCH$$
$$|$$
$$HOCH$$
$$|$$
$$HCOH$$
$$|$$
$$HCOH$$
$$|$$
$$CH_2.\underset{+}{N}H_2.CH_2.CH_2Cl$$

$. 2Cl^-$

$C_{10}H_{24}Cl_4N_2O_4$ Mol. wt: 378.1

1.3 Chemical and physical properties of the pure substance

(a) Description: White crystals from 80% ethanol

(b) Melting-point: 239-241°C (decomposition)

---

*This name is also used for the free base.

(c) __Optical rotation__: $[\alpha]_D^{20}$ + 18.46^O (1.8% in water)

(d) __Identity test__: A test is given in __British Pharmaceutical Codex__ (1973).

(e) __Solubility__: Soluble in water (1 part in 2);   slightly soluble in ethanol;   insoluble in chloroform and ether

(f) __Stability__: Aqueous solutions decompose to D-mannitol and $ClCH_2CH_2NHCH_3$ within 24 hours at 25°C (Narbutt-Mering, 1972).

1.4 Technical products and impurities

Mannomustine dihydrochloride is available in Europe in the form of tablets containing 50 mg active ingredient and in ampoules for intravenous injection containing 50 mg (Blacow, 1967; __Dictionnaire Vidal__, 1975; Pullom, 1968-69; Steinböck *et al.*, 1969).

2. Production, Use, Occurrence and Analysis

For important background information on this section, see preamble, p. 17.

Mannomustine

2.1 Production and use

Mannomustine can be prepared by treating 1,2,5,6-dianhydro-3,4-o-isopropylidine-D-mannitol with aziridine. The ethyleneimino derivative is then treated with hydrochloric acid to yield mannomustine dihydrochloride, which is converted to mannomustine by reaction with sodium hydroxide (Vargha *et al.*, 1957).

It has been tested as an antineoplastic agent, but it is not believed to be produced commercially.

2.2 Occurrence

Mannomustine is not known to occur in nature.

Mannomustine dihydrochloride

2.1 Production and use

Mannomustine dihydrochloride can be prepared by treating 1,6-ditosyl-

159

2,3,4,5-di-O-methylene-D-mannitol with ethanolamine to yield 1,6-di(β-hydroxyethylamino)-1,6-dideoxy-2,3,4,5-di-O-methylene-D-mannitol. Chlorination of the product with thionyl chloride gives mannomustine dihydrochloride (Toldy & Vargha, 1959).

This chemical is produced in Hungary and is used in human medicine for the treatment of malignant neoplasms, including breast and ovarian cancer, chronic leukaemias, lymphomas and myelomas. It is administered intravenously three times per week in doses of 1 mg/kg bw daily until a total dose of 500-1000 mg has been given (Brulé *et al.*, 1973). It is also available in tablet form for oral administration.

In Europe, studies have been made in laboratory animals on the immunosuppressive effects of mannomustine dihydrochloride for skin-grafting and kidney transplants (Mackiewicz *et al.*, 1969; Nemeth *et al.*, 1967); however, it is not known whether this chemical is sold commercially for use in this way in human medicine.

2.2 Occurrence

Mannomustine dihydrochloride is not known to occur in nature.

Mannomustine and mannomustine dihydrochloride

2.3 Analysis

The dihydrochloride can be estimated in blood by reaction with 4-(4'-nitrobenzyl)pyridine (NBP) at levels of 0.1-0.2 μmoles/ml (Körös *et al.*, 1964). A method of this type applicable to various biological fluids has been described by Truhaut *et al.* (1963), and a similar colorimetric method has been used for detection in various tissues (Maljtseva & Moskvitina, 1974). As little as 18 μg/ml mannomustine was detected using a 2% spray of NBP in acetone on silica gel plates (Sawicki & Sawicki, 1969). Reactions of mannomustine with various indicator dyes were tabulated by Palyi (1962); phenol red was found to be the most sensitive.

Paper (Palyi, 1962) and cellulose MN300 (Narbutt-Mering, 1972) have also been used as chromatographic media. A titration method for determining the purity of the drug is given in the British Pharmaceutical Codex (1973).

160

3. Biological Data Relevant to the Evaluation of Carcinogenic Risk to Man

3.1 Carcinogenicity and related studies in animals

(a) Intraperitoneal administration

Mouse: Groups of 30 AJ mice of both sexes, 4-6 weeks old, received i.p. injections of mannomustine dihydrochloride in water thrice weekly for 4 weeks (total doses, 2.2, 9, 36 and 144 mg/kg bw). At 39 weeks, 29, 24, 30 and 22 of the mice were surviving, and 12 (41%), 21 (87%), 22 (77%) and 20 (94%) had lung tumours, with 0.6, 1.8, 1.4 and 2.4 tumour nodules per mouse, respectively.   In 385 male and 392 female control mice receiving vehicle alone, 39.5% (male) and 31.4% (female) of the survivors developed lung tumours by 39 weeks, with 0.5 and 0.36 lung tumours per mouse, respectively.   In the same experiment, the potency of mannomustine dihydrochloride was reported to be 40 times less than that of uracil mustard on a molar basis (Shimkin et al., 1966).

A group of 100 male and 100 female C3 mice received i.p. injections of 2.5 mg/kg bw mannomustine dihydrochloride weekly for 52 weeks.   Lymphatic leukaemia occurred in 25% males and 23% females, and other leukaemias were observed in 7% males and 4% females.   Other tumours (unspecified) occurred in 18% males and 21% females.   In 200 controls of both sexes given 52 weekly injections of saline, the incidence of lymphatic leukaemia was 3.3% and those of other leukaemias and other tumours 0.5% and 9%, respectively (Németh, 1967).

(b) Intravenous administration

Rat: Fifty 100-day old male BR46 rats were given mannomustine dihydrochloride (4 mg/kg bw) by i.v. injection once weekly for 52 weeks. Among 37 surviving rats, malignant tumours were observed in 5 (14%) and benign tumours in 2 (5%) rats.   Three benign and 3 malignant tumours occurred in 85 controls (3.5%) (Schmähl, 1970).   In an almost identical experiment, 48 male BR46 rats, 100 days of age, were given 4 mg/kg bw mannomustine dihydrochloride by i.v. injection once weekly for 52 weeks.   Among 37 surviving rats, 2 (5%) developed benign tumours and 4 (11%), malignant tumours. Among 65 controls, 3 (5%) and 4 (6%) developed benign and malignant tumours, respectively (Schmähl & Osswald, 1970). [In neither study was the tumour incidence in treated animals statistically different from that in controls (P>0.05).]

3.2 Other relevant biological data

The i.p. LD_{50} for mannomustine dihydrochloride was 56-160 mg/kg bw in rats, depending on age and strain (Jeney et al., 1968; Raczynska-Bojanowska & Gasiorowska, 1966; Zsebok et al., 1965). The i.v. LD_{50} was 56-80 mg/kg bw in rats and 90, 50 and 50 mg/kg bw in mice, rabbits and dogs, respectively (Németh et al., 1958; Scherf et al., 1970; Schmähl, 1970; Schmähl & Osswald, 1970). Ruvidic (1962) reported an s.c. LD_{50} in mice of 120 mg/kg bw.

The principal toxic effect of mannomustine dihydrochloride is bone-marrow aplasia (Németh et al., 1958; Ruvidic, 1962); it is also immuno-suppressive (Scherf et al., 1970; Schmähl, 1971; Whitehouse et al., 1972), causes toxic liver damage at high doses (Lapis et al., 1958) and decreases renal functions (Bryukhanov, 1972). Mannomustine dihydrochloride prevented mitosis in the intestinal mucosa and in the ear skin but not in the corneal epithelium (Hadnagy et al., 1959).

Mannomustine dihydrochloride, ^{14}C-labelled in the ethylamino chain, was distributed heterogenously in the organs of 6-week old Wistar rats following its i.v. injection at a dose of 100 mg/kg bw. After 30 minutes, 2.1% of the applied radioactivity was found in the liver and 3.1% in the kidney. After 12 hours, these values had fallen to 0.28% and 0.21%, respectively; 63% of a dose of 8-15 mg/kg bw was excreted in the urine. No activity was detected in blood serum after 6 hours (Zsebok et al., 1965).

Liver RNA of mannomustine dihydrochloride-treated rats contained an unidentified bound product in the ion-exchange chromatography profiles of an HCl hydrolysate (Raczynska-Bojanowska & Gasiorowska, 1966). Incubation of the dihydrochloride with DNA at room temperature for 50 minutes changed the Tm point without changing the hyperchromicity of the DNA (Jeney et al., 1969).

Mannomustine dihydrochloride given to rats on the 13th day of pregnancy was not teratogenic, but the foetuses were only about half the normal size at birth (von Kreybig, 1970).

Mannomustine dihydrochloride induces chromosome aberrations in a fibrosarcoma rat cell line BGD$_2$ (Rimsa & Garzicic, 1970), in cultured human peripheral lymphocytes and in embryonic fibroblasts (Bochkov & Kuleshov, 1972; Mamaeva *et al.*, 1972).

In humans, approximately 50% of a single dose of 1 mg/kg bw mannomustine was removed from the blood within 20 minutes (Körös *et al.*, 1964).

3.3 Observations in man

No data were available to the Working Group.

4. Comments on Data Reported and Evaluation[1]

4.1 Animal data

Mannomustine administered as the dihydrochloride is carcinogenic in mice following its intraperitoneal injection, producing an increased incidence of leukaemia and a dose-related increase in the incidence of lung tumours.

4.2 Human data

No case reports or epidemiological studies were available to the Working Group.

---

[1]See also the section, "Animal Data in Relation to the Evaluation of Risk to Man" in the introduction to this volume, p. 15.

5. References

Blacow, N.W., ed. (1967) Martindale; The Extra Pharmacopoeia, 25th ed., London, The Pharmaceutical Press, p. 822

Bochkov, N.P. & Kuleshov, N.P. (1972) Age sensitivity of human chromosomes to alkylating agents. Mutation Res., 14, 345-353

British Pharmaceutical Codex (1973) London, The Pharmaceutical Press

Brulé, G., Eckhardt, S.J., Hall, T.C. & Winkler, A. (1973) Drug Therapy of Cancer, Geneva, World Health Organization, p. 43

Bryukhanov, V.M. (1972) Effect of Degranol on the secretory function of the kidneys. Farmakol. i Toksikol., 35, 46-48

Dictionnaire Vidal (1975) 51st ed., Paris, Office de Vulgarisation Pharmaceutique, pp. 405-406

Hadnagy, C., Gündisch, M., Gyergyay, F., Krepsz, I., Eperjessy, A., Kiss, A., Malatinszky, G.E., Kemény, G., Feszt, T. & Csegedi, J. (1959) Über die pharmakodynamische Wirkung von Degranol. Arch. int. Pharmacodyn., 120, 334-342

Jeney, A., Jr, Szabo, J. & Valyi-Nagy, T. (1968) Investigation on the mechanism of action of cytotoxic hexitols. II. The effect on the nucleic acid content of bone marrow in rats. Neoplasma, 15, 237-240

Jeney, A., Jr, Valyi-Nagy, T., Szabo, J. & Szabo, I. (1969) Investigation on the mode of action of the cytotoxic hexitols. III. Pharmaco-biochemical studies with Degranol. Neoplasma, 16, 151-159

Körös, Z., Hartai, F., Mâté-Wojcinska, U. & Sellei, C. (1964) Beiträge zum Wirkungsmechanismus des Degranols. Z. Krebsforsch., 66, 374-378

von Kreybig, T. (1970) Carcinogenese und Teratogenese: vergleichende Studien aus dem Aspekt der Teratologie. Arzneimittel-Forsch., 20, 591-601

Lapis, K., Németh, L., Békés, M. & Unger, E. (1958) Liver injury caused by antitumour drugs. Acta morph. Acad. Sci. hung., 8, 337-348

Mackiewicz, U., Mackiewicz, S. & Konys, J. (1969) Suppression of antibody synthesis and prolongation of skin allograft survival by alkylating agents. Ann. Immunol., 1, 59-67

Maljtseva, L.F. & Moskvitina, N.I. (1974) Distribution of Degranol in the rat organism. Vop. Onkol., 20, 75-77

Mamaeva, S.E., Fedortseva, R.F. & Goroshchenko, G.L. (1972) Effect of the alkylating agent Degranol on the chromosomes of cultured human lympho-cytes and embryonal fibroblasts. Tsitologia, 14, 89-96

Narbutt-Mering, A.B. (1972) Decomposition of chloroethylamine derivatives. Acta Pol. pharm., 29, 263-269

Nemeth, A., Kapros, K., Baradnay, G. & Simon, L. (1967) The immunosuppressive action of Degranol, vincaleukoblastine, dibromomannitol and mannitol-myleran in dogs with kidney homotransplants. Orv. Hetil., 108, 1257-1259

Németh, L. (1967) Vergleichende Untersuchung der karzinogenen Wirkung einiger zytostatischer Drogen und Röntgenstrahlen. Abstr. Europ. Cancer Meeting, Vienna, 3-5 July 1967, p. 71

Németh, L., Kellner, B. & Lapis, K. (1958) Comparative clinical and biological effects of alkylating agents. Ann. N.Y. Acad. Sci., 68, 879-888

Palyi, I. (1962) Detection of tumour-inhibiting mannitol derivatives by means of paper chromatography. J. Chromat., 9, 176-179

Pullom, E.N., ed. (1968-69) Mims Annual Compendium, London, Medical Publications Ltd, p. 74

Raczynska-Bojanowska, K. & Gasiorowska, I. (1966) The effect of nitrogen mustards on glutamate metabolism in rat liver mitochondria and Ehrlich ascites cells. Acta biochem. pol., 13, 113-120

Rimsa, D. & Garzicic, B. (1970) The effect of Degranol on tumour cell population *in vitro*. II. Action on the chromosomes of an established cell line *in vitro* during the isolation of the resistant strains. Genetika, 2, 71-79

Ruvidic, R. (1962) Désordres hématologiques et mortalité provoqués chez la souris par le dihydrochlorure de 1,6-bis-chloro-éthyl-amino-1,6-desoxy-D-mannitol. Effet de la transfusion de moelle osseuse. Rev. fr. Et. clin. biol., 7, 296-297

Sawicki, E. & Sawicki, C.R. (1969) Analysis of alkylating agents: application to air pollution. Ann. N.Y. Acad. Sci., 163, 895-920

Scherf, H.R., Krüger, C. & Karsten, C. (1970) Untersuchungen an Ratten über immunosuppressive Eigenschaften von Cytostatica unter besonderer Berücksichtigung der carcinogenen Wirkung. Arzneimittel-Forsch., 20, 1467-1470

Schmähl, D. (1970) Karzinogene Wirkungen von Krebschemotherapeutika. Onkol. Inform. Buil. Pulozkemie, 3, 5-8

Schmähl, D. (1971) Nebenwirkungen cytostatischer Therapie unter besonderer Berücksichtigung potentieller carcinogener Wirkungen. Internist, 12, 115-119

Schmähl, D. & Osswald, H. (1970) Experimentelle Untersuchungen über carcinogene Wirkungen von Krebs-Chemotherapeutica und Immunosuppressiva. Arzneimittel-Forsch., 20, 1461-1467

Shimkin, M.B., Weisburger, J.H., Weisburger, E.K., Gubareff, N.K. & Suntzeff, V. (1966) Bioassay of 29 alkylating chemicals by the pulmonary-tumor response in strain A mice. J. nat. Cancer Inst., 36, 915-935

Steinböck, R., Zekert, F. & Zimmermann, G. (1969) Austria-Codex, 1969/70, Vienna, Österreichischer Apotheker-Verlag, p. 214

Toldy, L. & Vargha, L. (1959) British Patent, 813,868, May 27, Gyogys-zeripari Kutato Intézet

Truhaut, R., Delacoux, E., Brulé, G. & Bohuon, C. (1963) Dosage des agents alcoylants dans les milieux biologiques. Méthode utilisant la réaction colorée avec la γ-(nitro-4-benzyl)-pyridine en milieu alcalin. Clin. chim. acta, 8, 235-245

Vargha, L., Toldy, L., Fehér, O. & Lendvai, S. (1957) Synthesis of new sugar derivatives of potential antitumour activity. I. Ethyleneimino- and 2-chloroethylamino-derivatives. J. chem. Soc., 805-809

Whitehouse, M.W., Droge, M.M. & Struck, R.F. (1972) Lymphocyte deactivation by cyclophosphamide metabolites and mannomustine. Proc. West. Pharmacol. Soc., 15, 195-199

Zsebok, Z., Torok, I. & Petranyi, G. (1965) Uber den Organtransport und Ausscheidungsmechanismus des 1,6-Bis(chloraethylamino)-1,6-desoxy-D-mannitol Dihydrochlorid. Strahlentherapie, 126, 111-118

MELPHALAN, MEDPHALAN & MERPHALAN

1. Chemical and Physical Data

Melphalan

1.1 Synonyms and trade names

Chem. Abstr. Reg. Serial No.:   148-82-3

Chem. Abstr. Name: 4-[Bis(2-chloroethyl)amino]-L-phenylalanine

L-3-{para-[Bis(2-chloroethyl)amino]phenyl}alanine;   CB 3025;   para-di(2-chloroethyl)amino-L-phenylalanine;   para-di(2-chloroethyl)amino-phenylalanine;   melfalan;   NSC-88-6;   phenylalanine mustard*;   L-phenylalanine mustard;   phenylalanine nitrogen mustard;   sarcolysin*;   L-sarcolysin;   sarcolysine*;   L-sarcolysine;   L-sarkolysin;   SK-15673

Alkeran

1.2 Chemical formula and molecular weight

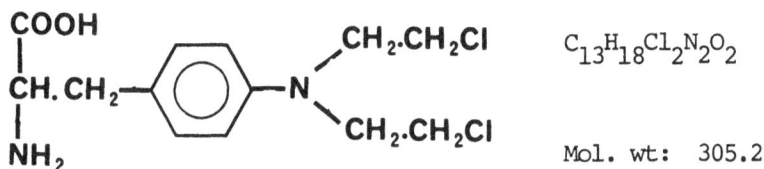

$C_{13}H_{18}Cl_2N_2O_2$

Mol. wt: 305.2

1.3 Chemical and physical properties of the pure substance

(a) Description: White, odourless powder

(b) Melting-point: Pure substance, 177°C (decomposition);   crystals from methanol, about 182°C (decomposition)

(c) Optical rotation: $[\alpha]_D^{22}$ +7.5° (1.33% in 1 N HCl)

or   -32.5° (0.67% in methanol)

---

*This name is also used for merphalan, which is a racemic mixture of the D and L isomers, medphalan and melphalan.

(<u>d</u>) <u>Spectroscopy data</u>: λ_{max} 260 nm; E_1^1 = 560 in aqueous solution
at pH 7

(<u>e</u>) <u>Identity test</u>:   Two colour tests are given in the <u>British</u>
<u>Pharmacopoeia</u> (British Pharmacopoeia Commission, 1973).

(<u>f</u>) <u>Solubility</u>:   Soluble in methanol (1 part in 150) and in ethanol,
propylene glycol, dilute mineral acid and alkali solutions and
2% carboxymethylcellulose;   practically insoluble in water;
insoluble in chloroform and ether

(<u>g</u>) <u>Stability</u>:   Hydrolyses in solution: half-life, 12.5 hours in
isotonic saline at 20°C and 1.8 hours at 37°C (Weale, 1964).
In 0.001 M NaCl (10 µg/ml) complete hydrolysis at 37°C takes
place in 3 hours, and at 100°C in 5 minutes (Chirigos & Mead,
1964).   Solutions at 4°C retained full activity for more than
24 hours (Espiner *et al*., 1962).

1.4   Technical products and impurities

Melphalan is available in the US as a USP grade in the form of tablets
containing 2 mg active ingredient (Kastrup, 1974).   Melphalan powder USP,
used to formulate the tablets, contains 93.0-100.5% melphalan, calculated
on the dried basis (US Pharmacopeial Convention, Inc., 1970).

In Western Europe, melphalan is available in tablets containing 2 and
5 mg and as injections equivalent to 100 mg anhydrous active ingredient in
1 ml solvent and 9 ml diluent (Bundesverband der pharmazeutischen Industrie,
1969;   <u>Dictionnaire Vidal</u>, 1975;   Pullom, 1968-69).

Medphalan

1.1   Synonyms and trade names

Chem. Abstr. Reg. Serial No.:   10345-94-8

Chem. Abstr. Name: 4-[Bis(2-chloroethyl)amino]-D-phenylalanine

(+)-3-{*para*-[Bis(2-chloroethyl)amino]phenyl}alanine;   D-3-{*para*-[bis-
(2-chloroethyl)amino]phenyl}alanine;   CB-3026;   *para*-di(2-chloroethyl)-
amino-D-phenylalanine;   medfalan;   NSC-35051;   D-phenylalanine mustard;
D-sarcolysine

1.2 Chemical formula and molecular weight

See melphalan.

1.3 Chemical and physical properties of the pure substance

(a) Description: White crystals from methanol

(b) Melting-point: About 182°C (decomposition)

(c) Optical rotation: $[\alpha]_D^{21}$ -7.5° (1.26% in 1 N HCl)

1.4 Technical products and impurities

Medphalan is not manufactured commercially.

Merphalan

1.1 Synonyms and trade names

Chem. Abstr. Reg. Serial No.: 531-76-0*

Chem. Abstr. Name: 4-[Bis(2-chloroethyl)amino]-DL-phenylalanine

3-{*para*-[Bis(2-chloroethyl)amino]phenyl}alanine; DL-3-{*para*-[bis-
(2-chloroethyl)amino]phenyl}alanine; CB-3307; *para*-di(2-chloroethyl)-
amino-DL-phenylalanine; merfalan; NSC-14210; phenylalanine mustard**;
DL-phenylalanine mustard; sarcolysin**; DL-sarcolysin; sarcolysine**;
DL-sarcolysine

Sarcoclorin

1.2 Chemical formula and molecular weight

See melphalan.

1.3 Chemical and physical properties of the pure substance

(a) Description: Needles from methanol

(b) Melting-point: 180-181°C (decomposition)

---

*Merphalan was originally allocated the Chem. Abstr. Reg. Serial No.
51-87-6; this has now been deleted, and the correct number is 531-76-0.

**This name is also used for melphalan, the L-isomeric constituent of
merphalan, a DL-racemic mixture.

(c) <u>Optical rotation</u>:   Optically inactive

1.4 Technical products and impurities

Although it is believed to be marketed in the USSR, no data were available.

2.   Production, Use, Occurrence and Analysis

For important background information on this section, see preamble, p. 17.

<u>Melphalan</u>

2.1 Production and use

Melphalan can be synthesized by treating *para*-nitro-L-phenylalanine ethyl ester with phthalic anhydride and then with hydrochloric acid to yield *para*-nitro-*N*-phthaloyl-L-phenylalanine ethyl ester. This product is then hydrogenated and treated with ammonia and ethylene oxide to give *para*-di-(2-hydroxyethyl)amino-*N*-α-phthaloyl-L-phenylalanine ethyl ester. Chlorination with phosphorous oxychloride followed by hydrolysis yields melphalan (Bergel & Stock, 1954, 1962).

Melphalan is produced in the UK by one company, which exports some of its production to the US and other countries. It is also produced in Italy (Chemical Information Services, Ltd, 1975). The amount exported to the US is not known, but it is estimated that total annual US sales of melphalan for use in human medicine are approximately 5 kg.

Melphalan is used in human medicine for the treatment of various malignant diseases, especially of multiple myeloma, malignant melanoma and adenocarcinomas of the ovary. The drug is usually administered in doses of 2-15 mg daily for a period of 2 or 3 weeks (British Pharmacopoeia Commission, 1973).

2.2 Occurrence

Melphalan is not known to occur in nature.

Medphalan

2.1 Production and use

Medphalan can be prepared by treating *para*-nitro-D-phenylalanine ethyl ester with phthalic anhydride and then with hydrochloric acid to yield *para*-nitro-*N*-phthaloyl-D-phenylalanine ethyl ester. This is hydrogenated and treated with ammonia and ethylene oxide to give *para*-di(2-hydroxyethyl)-amino-*N*-α-phthaloyl-D-phenylalanine ethyl ester. Chlorination with phosphorous oxychloride followed by hydrolysis yields medphalan (Bergel & Stock, 1954, 1962).

Medphalan has been tested as an antineoplastic agent in animals in the US and in Europe; however, melphalan and merphalan have been studied more extensively and have found use in human medicine (White, 1960).

2.2 Occurrence

Medphalan is not known to occur in nature.

Merphalan

2.1 Production and use

Merphalan was synthesized in the UK according to the method described for melphalan. At the same time, workers in the USSR synthesized merphalan by treating acetamido-*para*-aminobenzylmalonic ester with ethylene oxide and then with thionyl chloride to give acetamido-*para*-di(2-chloroethyl)amino-benzylmalonic ester, which was converted to merphalan by prolonged heating with hydrochloric acid (Larionov *et al.*, 1955).

Merphalan has been tested clinically as an antineoplastic agent in Europe and Japan (White, 1960) and is used as such in the USSR.

2.2 Occurrence

Merphalan is not known to occur in nature.

Melphalan, medphalan and merphalan

2.3 Analysis

The three stereoisomers react similarly with 4(4'-nitrobenzyl)pyridine; this can be used for their determination in plasma and urine and is sensitive

171

down to 5 µg/ml (Truhaut *et al.*, 1963). The method has been used to follow the reaction of phenylalanine mustards with blood *in vivo* and *in vitro* (Klatt *et al.*, 1960). Reactions with 2-nitroindan-1,2-dione (Kozlov & Bernshtein, 1968, 1970), sodium tetraphenylborane (De Carnevale-Bonino *et al.*, 1971) and *para*-N,N-dimethylaminobenzaldehyde (Kozlov & Bernshtein, 1968) have also been used to determine phenylalanine mustards. UV-spectrophotometry (Belousova, 1961), spectrofluorometry (detection limit, 0.05 µg/ml) (Chirigos & Mead, 1964) and titrimetry (British Pharmacopoeia Commission, 1973) can be used to determine the pure compounds in aqueous solution.

Phenylalanine mustards and their hydrolysis products have been separated by gas-liquid chromatography of the trimethylsilyl derivatives (Goras *et al.*, 1970) and by two-dimensional thin-layer chromatography on Kieselgel G (Walthier & Jeney, 1968).

3. Biological Data Relevant to the Evaluation of Carcinogenic Risk to Man

3.1 Carcinogenicity and related studies in animals

(a) Skin application

Mouse: Twenty-five S mice were given 10 weekly applications of a 0.1% w/v solution of medphalan in methanol (total dose, 3 mg). Thirty days after the start of treatment, croton oil was applied once weekly for 18 weeks. When the treatments overlapped medphalan and croton oil were applied alternately at 3-4-day intervals. By the end of the croton oil treatment 4/22 surviving mice had developed a total of 8 skin papillomas; and of 60 mice receiving various croton oil treatments 5/53 survivors had developed a total of 7 papillomas. [P>0.05]. At this time 18 of the survivors in the experimental group were killed, and 13 were found to have developed a total of 47 pulmonary adenomas (3.6 per mouse); in the control group 10/17 mice killed had developed a total of 17 lung adenomas (1.7 per mouse). In 1/3 of the remaining treated mice, a squamous-cell carcinoma of the skin developed 15 weeks after the end of the croton oil treatment.

An additional 25 mice received 10 weekly applications of a 0.01-0.1% w/v solution of melphalan in methanol (total dose, 1.44 mg), followed by croton oil treatment as above. The same controls as for medphalan were used. By the end of the treatment 2/19 survivors had developed a total of 7 skin papillomas. Of 13 survivors killed at this time 11 had a total of 57 pulmonary adenomas (5.1 per mouse). In 1/5 of the remaining treated animals an undifferentiated skin carcinoma developed 3 weeks after the end of treatment (Salaman & Roe, 1956). [The incidence of lung tumours seen in treated animals was not statistically different from that in controls.]

(b) Intraperitoneal administration

Mouse: Four groups of 60 A/J mice of both sexes, 4-6 weeks of age, were given i.p. injections of melphalan thrice weekly for 4 weeks (total doses, 0.27, 1.07, 4.27 and 17.1 mg/kg bw). At 39 weeks after the first dose there were 58, 56, 56 and 41 survivors, respectively, and 44%, 66%, 77% and 98% had developed lung tumours, with averages of 0.6, 1.0, 2.1 and 4.0 tumours per mouse. In 385 male and 392 female controls receiving vehicle only, the tumour incidences at 39 weeks were 39.5% (0.5 tumours/mouse) for males and 31.4% (0.36 tumours/mouse) for females. In the same experiment the potency of melphalan was reported to be about one quarter that of uracil mustard on a molar basis (Shimkin et al., 1966).

Two groups of 25 male and 25 female Swiss mice were given thrice weekly i.p. injections of 0.75 or 1.5 mg/kg bw melphalan for 6 months, followed by observation for a further 12 months, at which time the animals were killed. Lung tumours occurred in 11/44 males and 10/23 females, and lymphosarcomas were found in 13/44 males. The incidences for each tumour type were significantly greater in all cases than those in controls (P= 0.012, P=0.001 and P<0.001) (Weisburger et al., 1975).

Rat: Of 60 virgin female random-bred rats given single i.p. injections of 10 mg/kg bw merphalan, 9/33 survivors developed mammary fibroadenomas between 12 and 17 months. Of the controls, 30/40 animals survived, and no tumours of this type developed. In the same experiment 30 rats received single doses of 400 rads X-rays, and 8/19 survivors developed mammary fibroadenomas (Presnov & Jushkov, 1964).

Two groups of 25 male and 25 female Charles River CD rats were given thrice weekly i.p. injections of 0.9 or 1.8 mg/kg bw melphalan for 6 months, followed by observation for a further 12 months, at which time the animals were killed. Peritoneal sarcomas occurred in 11/20 males and 10/23 females, and these incidences were statistically greater than those in controls (P<0.001) (Weisburger *et al.*, 1975).

3.2 Other relevant biological data

The various biochemical properties of phenylalanine mustards, including their effect on the uptake of precursors into protein and nucleic acids and their action on several enzyme activities, have been reviewed (Connors, 1971; Wheeler, 1962).

The i.p. LD_{50} of merphalan in rats is 23 mg/kg bw (Cohn, 1957); it also inhibits bone-marrow haemopoiesis (Larionov *et al.*, 1955).

Two days after i.p. administration of 15 mg/kg bw β-^{14}C-merphalan to Walker carcinoma-bearing rats, the soluble protein fraction of kidney contained at least three times the specific activity compared to that of other tissues (e.g., blood, liver and Walker carcinoma), the level corresponding to no more than 60 μg merphalan/g protein (Cohn, 1957). After administration of ^{3}H-melphalan to Walker carcinoma-bearing rats, radioactivity was found in liver, spleen, kidney, intestine and Walker carcinoma and to a lesser extent in bone marrow, muscle, skin, testis and brain, but not in the DNA fraction of any of these tissues. Approximately 25% of the administered radioactivity was excreted in the urine during the first 48 hours (Milner *et al.*, 1965).

Merphalan was teratogenic in rats when given during the first 10 days of pregnancy, causing termination of pregnancy and various types of malformations (Aleksandrov, 1966). It exerts immunosuppressive effects in mice (Fontalin *et al.*, 1970; Kazaryan, 1970).

Melphalan produces structural aberrations of the chromatid and chromosome types in bone-marrow cells of treated Wistar rats (Wantzin & Jensen, 1973) and chromatid-type aberrations in peripheral blood lymphocytes taken from cancer patients (Sharpe, 1971).

Merphalan is mutagenic, inducing streptomycin-independent reversions in strain Sd-4-73 of *Escherichia coli* (Szybalski, 1958).

After its administration to cancer patients by perfusion, 60% <u>merphalan</u> was removed from the blood within 45 minutes. It reacts rapidly with heparinized blood: 40% of the administered dose had reacted within 45 minutes at 37°C *in vitro* (Klatt *et al.*, 1960).

DNA synthesis was inhibited in the myeloma cells of cancer patients given 2 mg <u>melphalan</u> per day (Hiroshi *et al.*, 1972).

3.3 Observations in man

Karchmer *et al.* (1974) and Kyle *et al.* (1975) have summarized 28 case reports of acute leukaemia which developed in patients administered alkylating agents, combined in some cases with irradiation, for the treatment of myeloma. In 19 cases <u>melphalan</u> was the only form of chemotherapy, although in 7 cases (and possibly in 2 others) irradiation was also given. The dose of melphalan was 2-6 mg/day for 15-102 months, and the leukaemias (all of myeloid or monocytic type) developed 15-114 months (median, 45 months) after diagnosis of myeloma. Another patient, reported by Holt *et al.* (1972), developed a typical myelocytic leukaemia while in remission from myeloma after having received 1.2 g melphalan over a 4-year period. Three cases of reticulosarcoma of a plasma-cell type involving non-lymphoreticular tissues have also been described in patients with myeloma who had been treated with melphalan, although in one case radiotherapy had been given and in one other case cyclophosphamide had also been administered (Holt & Robb-Smith, 1973; Levin *et al.*, 1967; River & Schorr, 1966). A bronchogenic carcinoma has been reported in a myeloma patient treated with melphalan (Scheidegger, 1972).

4. Comments on Data Reported and Evaluation

4.1 Animal data

Melphalan is carcinogenic in mice and rats following its intraperitoneal injection, producing lymphosarcomas and a dose-related increase in lung tumours in mice and peritoneal sarcomas in rats. Merphalan (a mixture of medphalan and melphalan) produced an increased incidence of mammary fibroadenomas in rats following its intraperitoneal injection in single doses.

175

4.2 Human data

The available case reports suggest that the incidence of acute leukaemia is increased in myeloma patients treated with melphalan.

5. References

Aleksandrov, V.A. (1966) Peculiarities of the pathogenic action of sarcolysine on rat embryogenesis. Dokl. Akad. Nank. SSSR, 171, 746-749

Belousova, A.K. (1961) Spectrophotometric determination of some chloro-ethylamines and products of their hydrolysis. Vop. Onkol., 7, 54-63

Bergel, F. & Stock, J.A. (1954) Cyto-active amino-acid and peptide deriva-tives. I. Substituted phenylalanines. J. chem. Soc., 2409-2417

Bergel, F. & Stock, J.A. (1962) p-[Bis(2-chloroethyl)amino]phenylalanine. US Patent, 3,032,584, May 1, National Research Development Corp.

British Pharmacopoeia Commission (1973) British Pharmacopoeia, London, HMSO, p. 284

Bundesverband der pharmazeutischen Industrie (1969) Rote Liste, Frankfurt, p. 34

Chemical Information Services, Ltd (1975) Directory of Western European Chemical Producers, 1975/76, Oceanside, NY

Chirigos, M.A. & Mead, J.A.R. (1964) Experiments on determination of melphalan by fluorescence. Interaction with protein and various solutions. Analyt. Biochem., 7, 259-268

Cohn, P. (1957) The distribution of radioactivity in tissues of the rat following the administration of a nitrogen mustard derivative (p-di-(2-chloroethyl)amino-DL-phenyl(β-^{14}C)alanine. Brit. J. Cancer, 11, 258-267

Connors, T.A. (1971) Effects of drugs on structure, biosynthesis and cata-bolism of nucleic acids, proteins, carbohydrates and lipids. Nucleic acids and protein. Drugs which combine chemically with nucleic acids: alkylating agents. In: Bacq, Z.M. et al., eds, Fundamentals of Biochemical Pharmacology, Elmsford, New York, Pergamon Press, pp. 461-475

De Carnevale Bonino, R.C.D., Dobrecky, J. & Guerello, L.O. (1971) Estimation of cytostatics using sodium tetraphenylborane and volumetric analysis in a non-aqueous medium. Rev. farm. (B. Aires), 113, 15-19

Dictionnaire Vidal (1975) 51st ed., Paris, Office de Vulgarisation Pharmaceutique, p.55

Espiner, H.J., Vowles, K.D.J. & Walker, R.M. (1962) Cancer chemotherapy by intra-arterial infusion. A preliminary report concerning tumours of the head and neck. Lancet, i, 177-181

Fontalin, L.N., Pevnitskii, L.A., Solov'ev, V.V., Kazaryan, K.A. & Filitis, L.N. (1970) Analysis of immunodepressive activity of some chemical agents and their utilization for creating immunological tolerance in the post-natal period. Vestn. Akad. med. Nauk, 25, 75-86

Goras, J.T., Knight, J.B., Iwamoto, R.H. & Lim, P. (1970) Gas-liquid chromatographic determination of melphalan. J. pharm. Sci., 59, 561-563

Hiroshi, H., Kzuo, N. & Kiyoyasu, N. (1972) Kinetic studies on human myeloma cells following melphalan administration. Acta haemat. jap. 34, 614

Holt, J.M. & Robb-Smith, A.H. (1973) Multiple myeloma: development of plasma cell sarcoma during apparently successful chemotherapy. J. clin. Path., 26, 649-659

Holt, J.M., Robb-Smith, A.H.T., Callender, S.T. & Spriggs, A.I. (1972) Multiple myeloma: Development of alternative malignancy following successful chemotherapy. Brit. J. Haemat., 22, 633

Karchmer, R.K., Amare, M., Larsen, W.E., Mallouk, A.G. & Caldwell, G.G. (1974) Alkylating agents as leukaemogens in multiple myeloma. Cancer, 33, 1103-1107

Kastrup, E.K., ed. (1974) Facts and Comparisons, St Louis, Missouri, Facts & Comparisons Inc.

Kazaryan, K.A. (1970) Immunodepressive activity of some radiomimetics during immunization of mice with sheep erythrocytes. Byull. éksp. Biol. Med., 69, 87-91

Klatt, O., Griffin, A.C. & Stehlin, J.S., Jr (1960) Method for determination of phenylalanine mustard and related alkylating agents in blood. Proc. Soc. exp. Biol. (N.Y.), 104, 629-631

Kozlov, K.E. & Bernshtein, V.N. (1968) Qualitative and quantitative analysis of drugs of the bis(2-chloroethyl)amine group. Aktual. Vop. Farm., 61-65

Kozlov, K.E. & Bernshtein, V.N. (1970) Qualitative and quantitative analysis of medicinal preparations: derivatives of bis(2-chloroethyl)amine. Farmatsiya (Moscow), 19, 34-35

Kyle, R.A., Pierre, R.V. & Bayrd, E.D. (1975) Multiple myeloma and acute leukemia associated with alkylating agents. Arch. intern. Med., 135, 185-192

Larionov, L.F., Khokhlov, A.S., Shkodinskaja, E.N., Vasina, O.S., Troosheikina, V.I. & Novikova, M.A. (1955) Studies on the anti-tumour activity of p-di(2-chloroethyl)aminophenylalanine (sarcolysine). Lancet, i, 169-171

Levin, H.A., Freeman, R.G., Smith, F.E. & Lane, M. (1967) Multiple extra-medullary plasmacytomas. Arch. Derm., 96, 456-461

Milner, A.N., Klatt, O., Young, S.E. & Stehlin, J.S., Jr (1965) The biochemical mechanism of action of L-phenylalanine mustard. I. Distribution of L-phenylalanine mustard-H^3 in tumour bearing rats. Cancer
Res., 25, 259-264

Presnov, M.A. & Jushkov, S.F. (1964) The development of mastopathy and
fibroadenoma in the rat mammary gland after intraabdominal sarcolysin
injection. Vop. Onkol., 10, 66-72

Pullom, E.N., ed. (1968-69) Mims Annual Compendium, London, Medical
Publications Ltd, p. 92

River, G.L. & Schorr, W.F. (1966) Malignant skin tumors in multiple myeloma.
Arch. Derm., 93, 432-438

Salaman, M.H. & Roe, F.J.C. (1956) Further tests for tumour-initiating
activity: N,N-di-(2-chloroethyl)-p-aminophenylbutyric acid (CB 1348)
as an initiator of skin tumour formation in the mouse. Brit. J. Cancer,
10, 363-377

Scheidegger, S. (1972) Lungenfibrose, rezidivierende Vasculitis und multi-
zentrisches Lungencarcinom nach cytostatischer Therapie mit Alkeran.
Verh. dtsch. Ges. Path., 56, 364-368

Sharpe, H.B.A. (1971) Observations on the effect of therapy with nitrogen
mustard or a derivative on chromosomes of human peripheral blood
lymphocytes. Cell Tissue Kinet., 4, 501-504

Shimkin, M.B., Weisburger, J.H., Weisburger, E.K., Gubareff, N.K. & Suntzeff,
V. (1966) Bioassay of 29 alkylating chemicals by the pulmonary tumor
response in strain A mice. J. nat. Cancer Inst., 36, 915-935

Szybalski, W. (1958) Special microbiological systems. II. Observations
on chemical mutagenesis in microorganisms. Ann. N.Y. Acad. Sci., 76,
475-489

Truhaut, R., Delacoux, E., Brule, G. & Bohuon, D. (1963) Dosage des agents
alcoylants dans les milieux biologiques. Méthode utilisant la réaction
colorée avec la γ-(nitro-4-benzyl)-pyridine en milieu alcalin.
Clin. chim. acta, 8, 235-245

US Pharmacopeial Convention, Inc. (1970) The US Pharmacopeia, 18th rev.,
Easton, Pa , Mack, pp. 393-394

Walthier, J. & Jeney, A. (1968) Thin-layer chromatography for biological
alkylating agents. Acta pharm. hung., 38, 236-244

Wantzin, G.L. & Jensen, M.K. (1973) The induction of chromosome abnormalities
by melphalan in rat bone-marrow cells. Scand. J. Haemat., 11, 135-139

Weale, F.E. (1964) Ice-cooled melphalan for regional infusion. Lancet, i, 23-24

Weisburger, J.H., Griswold, D.P., Jr, Prejean, J.D., Casey, A.E., Wood, H.B., Jr & Weisburger, E.K. (1975) The carcinogenic properties of some of the principal drugs used in clinical cancer chemotherapy. Recent Results Cancer Res. (in press)

Wheeler, G.P. (1962) Studies related to the mechanism of action of cyto-toxic alkylating agents: A review. Cancer Res., 22, 651-687

White, F.R. (1960) New agent data summaries. Sarcolysin and related compounds. Cancer Chemother. Rep., 6, 61-93

MUSTARD GAS

1. Chemical and Physical Data

1.1 Synonyms and trade names

Chem. Abstr. Reg. Serial No.:   505-60-2

Chem. Abstr. Name: 1,1'-Thiobis(2-chloroethane)

Bis(2-chloroethyl)sulphide;   bis(β-chloroethyl)sulphide;   1-chloro-2-(β-chloroethylthio)ethane;   2,2'-dichlorodiethyl sulphide;   di-2-chloroethyl sulphide;   β,β'-dichloroethyl sulphide;   Schwefel-Lost;   S-lost;   S mustard;   sulphur mustard;   sulphur mustard gas;   yellow cross liquid

Yperite

1.2 Chemical formula and molecular weight

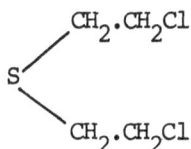

$$S \Big\langle \begin{array}{l} CH_2.CH_2Cl \\ CH_2.CH_2Cl \end{array} \qquad\qquad C_4H_8Cl_2S \qquad Mol.\ wt:\ 159.1$$

1.3 Chemical and physical properties of the pure substance

(a) Description: Colourless, odourless, oily liquid;   forms prisms on cooling

(b) Melting-point: 13-14°C

(c) Boiling-point: 215-217°C at 760 mm Hg;   108°C at 14 mm Hg; 98°C at 10 mm Hg

(d) Density: d_4^{20} 1.274 (liquid); d^{13} 1.338 (solid)

(e) Refractive index: n_D^{20} 1.531

(f) Solubility: Sparingly soluble in water (0.68 g/l at 25°C); soluble in fat, fat solvents and other common organic solvents (Seidell, 1941;   Stecher, 1968)

181

(g) <u>Volatility</u>: Volatile with steam; vapour pressure at $0^{\circ}C$ is 0.025 mm Hg, and 0.09 mm Hg at $30^{\circ}C$

(h) <u>Stability</u>: Hydrolysed in aqueous solution ($t\frac{1}{2}$, 5 minutes at $37^{\circ}C$). The products of hydrolysis are thiodiglycol and hydrochloric acid (Berenblum, 1935).

(i) <u>Reactivity</u>: Reacts with sulphhydryl and imidazole groups (Dawson *et al.*, 1959). Its reaction with bleach and chlorine provides a method of decontamination.

1.4 <u>Technical products and impurities</u>

Mustard gas is believed to be produced in small quantities by manufacturers of laboratory chemicals.

2. <u>Production, Use, Occurrence and Analysis</u>

For important background information on this section, see preamble, p. 17.

2.1 <u>Production and use</u>

Mustard gas may have been synthesized by Despretz (Despretz, 1822), but large quantities were not manufactured until World War I: by 1919, US production had increased to approximately 18,000 kg per day. At that time mustard gas was synthesized in the US by reacting ethylene with sulphur monochloride at $30-35^{\circ}C$. In Germany it was produced by treating ethylene first with hypochlorous acid and then with sodium sulphide, to yield β,β'-dihydroxyethyl sulphide. This product was then heated with hydrochloric acid, yielding mustard gas (Jackson, 1936).

Mustard gas was used as a vesicant in chemical warfare during World War I and in Ethiopia in 1936 (United Nations, 1969). Although no further military use was reported, production and stockpiling of this chemical continued, especially during World War II (Rose, 1968) and stocks may still have existed in the US as recently as 1974 (Anon., 1974).

Mustard gas has been tested as an antineoplastic agent (Huntress *et al.*, 1963), but its clinical use as a tumour inhibitor has been minimal. It is used as a model compound in biological studies on alkylating agents.

182

2.2 Occurrence

For some time after July 1917, much of the French soil in the region of battle lines was contaminated with mustard gas (Case & Lea, 1955). The average and maximum atmospheric concentrations likely to have been produced under military conditions, in the area of falling shells, have been esti-mated to be 3 and 5 ppm, respectively (Thorpe, 1974).

2.3 Analysis

Gas chromatographic methods are available for the determination of mustard gas (Albro & Fishbein, 1970; Casselmann *et al.*, 1973). It can also be estimated in air at levels of 0.5-1 µg/l air using detection tubes containing 4-(4'-nitrobenzyl)pyridine complexes with bivalent mercury, nickel and magnesium salts and using purified activated silica gel as carrier (Kratochvil & Martinek, 1969).

3. Biological Data Relevant to the Evaluation of Carcinogenic Risk to Man

3.1 Carcinogenicity and related studies in animals

(a) Inhalation and/or intratracheal administration

Mouse: A group of 40 male and 40 female A mice, 2-3 months of age, was exposed for 15 minutes to vapours from 100 cm^3 mustard gas in an 8-litre dessicator; 40 male and 40 female controls were exposed to air alone. Four months after exposure 30 test and 32 control mice were killed, and the incidences of lung tumours were found to be 9/30 and 6/32, respectively. All other surviving animals were killed after 11 months of exposure, and 33/67 mice exposed to mustard gas (including those already mentioned) had lung tumours (unspecified), compared with 21/77 controls. The numbers of tumours per mouse were 0.66 in the exposed group and 0.31 in the controls. The difference in incidence compared with that in controls is reported to be highly significant (P<0.01) (Heston & Levillain, 1953).

(b) Subcutaneous and/or intramuscular administration

Mouse: Three groups of 2-3-month old mice, comprising 16 C3H mice of both sexes, 10 female C3Hf mice and 30 A mice of both sexes, were given 5-6

weekly s.c. injections of 0.05 ml of a 0.05% solution of mustard gas in
olive oil and were observed until natural death (average survival times,
7 months in A males to 15 months in C3Hf females). Fibrosarcomas at the
injection site were observed in 1/8 C3H males, 2/9 C3Hf females and 1/14
A males 10-14 months after the beginning of treatment. Mammary tumours
were also observed in 2 female C3Hf mice, in 8/8 treated C3H females and in
1/12 treated A females; in a concurrent study mammary tumours were reported
to have occurred in 2/100 female C3Hf controls, in 7/8 C3H controls, and
in 0/14 A controls. In a second experiment, a rhabdomyosarcoma occurred
after 15 months in 1/24 C3H males, and local sarcomas were observed in
2/38 C3Hf males about 15 months after the start of treatment. No subcutaneous sarcomas occurred in 60 non-injected C3H or C3Hf male controls nor
in male and female C3H and A controls injected with olive oil (Heston,
1953). [P>0.05].

   (c) Intravenous administration

   Mouse: A group of 15 male and 15 female A mice, 2 months old, was
injected intravenously on alternate days with 0.25 ml of a 1:10 dilution
of a saturated solution of mustard gas in water (0.06-0.07%) for a total
of 4 injections. All survivors were killed at the age of 6 months, and
14/15 (93%) treated mice had developed pulmonary tumours (2.6 tumours/
mouse), compared with 15/28 (61%) controls (0.9 tumours/mouse). In a
second experiment, in which a slightly lower dose of mustard gas was
administered intravenously to 24 males and 24 females, pulmonary tumours
were found in 32/47 (68%) treated survivors (1.09 tumours/mouse) at the age
of 6 months, compared with 6/46 (13%) in controls (0.13 tumours/mouse)
(Heston, 1950). [P<0.001].

3.2 Other relevant biological data

   The i.v. LD$_{50}$ in rats is 0.7 mg/kg bw (Stecher, 1968).

   Mustard gas inhibited the carcinogenic action of coal-tar on mouse
skin (Berenblum, 1935).

   Following i.v. injection of 5 mg/kg bw ^{35}S-labelled mustard gas into
rabbits, the radioactivity was rapidly diffused throughout the body; about
one-fifth of the activity was excreted in the urine within 12 hours; excre-

tion *via* the bile was noted; and the liver, lungs and kidneys were the main organs in which radioactivity was retained (Boursnell *et al.*, 1946). In mice and rats given 1-5 mg/kg bw ^{35}S-labelled mustard gas by i.v. injection, very small amounts of radioactivity were found in the expired air (0.05%) and faeces (6%) of rats, the majority of the injected dose being excreted in the urine within 72 hours. The main urinary metabolites were thiodiglycol and conjugates (15%), glutathione-bis-β-chloroethylsulphide conjugates (45%), glutathione-bis-β-chloroethylsulphone conjugates (7%) and bis-β-chloroethylsulphone and conjugates (8%). Very small amounts of cysteine conjugates were also present (Davison *et al.*, 1961). I.p. injection of 1 mg ^{35}S-mustard gas in rats resulted in the urinary excretion of bis-cysteinylethylsulphone and small amounts (15%) of thiodiglycol metabolites (Roberts & Warwick, 1963).

Mustard gas reacts *in vivo* with proteins and nucleic acids of the lung, liver and kidney of A/J mice (Abell, 1964). The perfusion of lungs isolated from dogs showed that equilibrium between the blood and tissues was reached after 5 minutes and that 14% of the activity was retained in the lung (Pierpont & Davison, 1962).

Mustard gas, at low concentrations, has been shown to inhibit DNA synthesis in *E. coli* bacteria (Lawley & Brookes, 1965), in HeLa cells (Crathorn & Roberts, 1966; Roberts *et al.*, 1971a), in L-cells (Reid & Walker, 1969) and in HeLa and Chinese hamster cells (Roberts *et al.*, 1971b). 7-Hydroxyethylthioethylguanine and di(guanin-7-yl)ethyl sulphide have been identified in the cross-linking of the DNA double helix (Lawley & Brookes, 1965; Reid & Walker, 1969). Cell recovery after enzymatically mediated removal of such cross-links has been demonstrated in both bacterial and mammalian cell systems.

Mustard gas was the first chemical reported to induce mutations and chromosome rearrangements in *Drosophila melanogaster* (Auerbach & Robson, 1946) and mutations in specific DNA regions (r-RNA coding bb locus) (Fahmy & Fahmy, 1971). It induces chromosome aberrations in cultured rat lymphosarcoma cell lines (Scott *et al.*, 1974); and in a host-mediated assay in male BDF$_1$ mice, using murine leukaemia L5178Y/Asn$^-$ cell line as indicator, it induced both chromosome aberrations and reverse mutations to asparagine

independence after single s.c. doses of 100 mg/kg bw. Similar results
were obtained with the same cell line tested *in vitro* (Capizzi *et al.*,
1973). Dominant lethal mutations in adult male virgin rats were induced
after exposure to mustard gas at 0.1 mg/m^3 of air for 52 weeks (Rozmiarek
et al., 1973).

Two terminal cancer patients given i.v. doses of 5 mg (0.1 mg/kg bw)
^{35}S-labelled mustard gas in ethanol excreted 23% of the radioactivity in
urine within 24 hours and 27% after 48 hours. The urinary metabolites
were the same as those found in rat and mouse urine, as judged by similari-
ties in column chromatographic eluant patterns (Davison *et al.*, 1961).

3.3 Observations in man

Case & Lea (1955) examined the mortality records from 1930-1952 of
1267 war pensioners who suffered from mustard gas poisoning during 1917-
1918. The results were compared with those obtained from two other groups:
(a) 1421 war pensioners who suffered from chronic bronchitis, but who had
never been exposed to mustard gas and (b) 1114 war pensioners who were
wounded but who had not been poisoned by mustard gas. In both the mustard
gas and chronic bronchitis groups an excess mortality was found compared
with that expected from the general male population mortality rates in
England and Wales. This was mainly accounted for by an excess of deaths
from chronic bronchitis. Mortality from cancer of the lung and pleura was
also greater in these two groups and to an equal extent (in both, 29
observed, compared to 14 expected) but not in the amputation group (13,
compared to 16 expected). There were no significant differences in any of
the three groups between observed and expected numbers of cancers involving
sites other than the lung and pleura. It was noted that almost all of
those in the mustard gas group also suffered from chronic bronchitis, from
which there was a high mortality (217, compared to 21 expected). The
authors concluded that the increased risk of lung and pleural cancer could
not be attributed to mustard gas poisoning but appeared to be associated
in some way with chronic bronchitis. No account could be taken of smoking
habits in this study. However, it may be relevant that Dorn (1958, quoted
in Norman, 1975) has shown that a significantly higher proportion of men
injured by mustard gas had given up smoking before the age of 40. It is

possible, therefore, that the presence of a greater proportion of chronic smokers in the bronchitis group resulted in a greater mortality from lung cancer due to smoking than in the mustard gas group, and that this evidence was masked by a carcinogenic effect of the gas.

Mortality records from 1919-1955 were examined for 2718 American soldiers exposed to mustard gas during 1917-1918, for 1855 soldiers who had pneumonia during the influenza epidemic of 1918 but who had not been exposed to mustard gas and for 2578 wounded soldiers with no history of mustard gas poisoning or of pneumonia. Differences in mortality in the three groups were seen only in the second decade (1930-39) of the follow-up, at which time the mustard gas group suffered a higher mortality, mainly from pneumonia and tuberculosis. There were 36 deaths from lung cancer (1.3%) in the mustard gas group, compared with 14 (0.8%) in the pneumonia group and 26 (1%) in the war-wounded group. Differences in the incidence of chronic bronchitis were noted (65%, 35% and 20% in the mustard gas, pneumonia and wounded groups, respectively) and in the proportion of men who had stopped smoking. A comparison of the numbers of deaths from all respiratory cancers with the expected numbers, calculated from US mortality rates, showed the following ratios of observed to expected cases: mustard gas, 39:26 (1.47); pneumonia, 15:18 (0.81); and war-wounded, 30:26 (1.15). These data suggest that mustard gas exposure is associated with an increased risk of respiratory cancer, but that the extent of the increase is not large (Beebe, 1960). The results of a further study involving an additional 10 years of follow-up of these groups did not alter the original conclusion (Norman, 1975).

A stronger association between mustard gas exposure and respiratory cancer is indicated by the experience of workers in a Japanese factory which manufactured this gas from 1929-1945 and on a large scale in the period 1937-1944. Protective measures were neither fully effective nor generally applied, and the working environment attained mustard gas concentrations of 0.05-0.07 mg/l. The first suspicion of an increased risk of cancer came in 1952 from a death from bronchial cancer of a 30-year old male who had been occupationally exposed to mustard gas for 16 months from 1941 (Yamada *et al.*, 1953). Four cases of squamous-cell carcinomas of the larynx and one carcinoma *in situ* affecting the same site were reported in Japanese workers

17-24 years after occupational exposure to mustard gas for 5-13 years. Furthermore, of 97 deaths in exposed workers, respiratory cancer accounted for 60% (12) of deaths from malignant tumours (20) in the period 1946-1957 (Yamada *et al.*, 1957).

Yamada (1963) examined a series of 172 deaths in former workers in this factory and found that 48 (27.9%) were from cancer; of these 28 (16.3%) were of the respiratory tract and oropharynx. Twenty-three were examined histologically, and 16 were found to be squamous-cell and 7, undifferentiated cancers occurring at the following sites: tongue (1), sinuses (1), pharynx (3), larynx (6), trachea (1) and bronchus (11). Of 5030 deaths in non-exposed inhabitants of the same area, 406 (8.1%) were from cancer, of which only 19 (0.4%) involved the respiratory tract.

Extending the study for the period 1952-1967, Wada *et al.* (1968) compared the observed numbers of deaths to those expected on the basis of Japanese mortality experience. Among 495 workers who had manufactured mustard gas, 33 had died from cancers of the respiratory tract, compared to 0.9 expected. Of 960 male employees not engaged in the production of the gas, only 3 were known to have died since 1952 from respiratory tract cancers, compared to 1.8 expected. Although there was evidence of preferential reporting of deaths in the gas-exposed group, the excess of respiratory tract cancers in this group was substantial.

Another study has recently been reported of workers in Germany engaged in the production, testing and destruction of mustard gas and nitrogen mustard, mainly during the period 1935-45. The factory employed 878 workers, less than half of whom worked in close contact with mustard gas, nitrogen mustard or with a mixture of the two. In addition, there was some limited exposure in the factory to bromoacetone, phosgene, chloropicrine and organic arsenicals. Of that relatively small population of workers exposed to the gas or to nitrogen mustard and for whom records were available, there were 85 deaths in the years 1951-1972 and of these 32 were due to cancer. An excess of certain cancers over those expected from the mortality rates for Lower Saxony was found, but this was significant only in the case of bronchial carcinomas (11, compared to 5 expected). It must be noted that the restriction of the study to workers with available medical records raises the possibility that the proportion with cancer may have been inflated, since medical or autopsy records would more likely have been preserved for workers with cancer (Weiss & Weiss, 1975).

4. Comments on Data Reported and Evaluation

4.1 Animal data

Mustard gas is carcinogenic in mice, the only species tested, following their exposure to its vapours or following its intravenous injection, inducing an increase in the incidence of lung tumours. Following its sub-cutaneous injection in mice, it produced a low incidence of sarcomas at the site of injection.

4.2 Human data

There is evidence of an increased incidence of cancers of the respiratory tract in men exposed to mustard gas.

5. References

Abell, C.W. (1964) The *in vivo* reaction of sulphur mustard with protein and ribonucleic acid isolated from the tissues of A/J mice. Proc. Amer. Assoc. Cancer Res, 5, 1

Albro, P.W. & Fishbein, L. (1970) Gas chromatography of sulphur mustard and its analogues. J. Chromat., 46, 202-203

Anon. (1974) House stirs up chemical warfare issues. Chemical and Engineering News, August 19, pp. 19-20

Auerbach, C. & Robson, J.M. (1946) Chemical production of mutations. Nature (Lond.), 157, 302

Beebe, G.W. (1960) Lung cancer in World War I veterans: possible relation to mustard gas injury and 1918 influenza epidemic. J. nat. Cancer Inst., 25, 1231-1252

Berenblum, I. (1935) Experimental inhibition of tumour induction by mustard gas and other compounds. J. Path. Bact., 40, 549-558

Boursnell, J.C., Cohen, J.A., Dixon, M., Francis, G.E., Greville, G.D., Needham, D.M. & Wormall, A. (1946) Studies on mustard gas ($\beta\beta'$-dichloro-diethylsulphide) and some related compounds. V. The fate of injected mustard gas (containing radioactive sulphur) in the animal body. Biochem. J., 40, 756-764

Capizzi, R.L., Smith, W.J., Field, R. & Papirmeister, B. (1973) A host-mediated assay for chemical mutagens using the L5178Y/Asn murine leukemia. Mutation Res., 21, 6

Case, R.A.M. & Lea, A.J. (1955) Mustard gas poisoning, chronic bronchitis and lung cancer. An investigation into the possibility that poisoning by mustard gas in the 1914-18 war might be a factor in the production of neoplasia. Brit. J. prev. soc. Med., 9, 62-72

Casselmann, A.A., Gibson, N.C.C. & Bannard, R.A.B. (1973) A rapid, sensitive, gas-liquid chromatographic method for the analysis of bis(2-chloroethyl)-sulfide collected from air in hydrocarbon solvents. J. Chromat., 78, 317-322

Crathorn, A.R. & Roberts, J.J. (1966) Mechanism of the cytotoxic action of alkylating agents in mammalian cells and evidence for the removal of alkylated groups from deoxyribonucleic acid. Nature (Lond.), 211, 150-153

Davison, C., Rozman, R.S. & Smith, P.K. (1961) Metabolism of bis-β-chloro-ethyl sulfide (sulfur mustard gas). Biochem. Pharmacol., 7, 65-74

Dawson, R.M.C., Elliott, D.C., Elliott, W.H. & Jones, K.M., eds (1959) Data for Biochemical Research, Oxford, Clarendon Press

Despretz, M. (1822) Des composés triples du chlore. Ann. chem. Phys., 21, 438

Fahmy, O.G. & Fahmy, M.J. (1971) Mutability at specific euchromatic and heterochromatic loci with alkylating and nitroso compounds in Drosophila melanogaster. Mutation Res., 13, 19-34

Heston, W.E. (1950) Carcinogenic action of the mustards. J. nat. Cancer Inst., 11, 415-423

Heston, W.E. (1953) Occurrence of tumors in mice injected subcutaneously with sulfur mustard and nitrogen mustard. J. nat. Cancer Inst., 14, 131-140

Heston, W.E. & Levillain, W.D. (1953) Pulmonary tumors in strain A mice exposed to mustard gas. Proc. Soc. exp. Biol. (N.Y.), 82, 457-460

Huntress, W.T., Goodridge, T.H. & Bratzel, R.P. (1963) Survey of sulfur mustards. Cancer Chemother. Rep., 26, 323-338

Jackson, K.E. (1936) The history of mustard gas. Tennessee Acad. Sci. J., 11, 98-106

Kratochvil, V. & Martinek, J. (1969) Neues Verfahren zum Nachweis von Yperit. Chemické Zvesti, 23, 382-390

Lawley, P.D. & Brookes, P. (1965) Molecular mechanism of the cytotoxic action of difunctional alkylating agents and of resistance to this action. Nature (Lond.), 206, 480-483

Norman, J.E. (1975) Lung cancer mortality in World War I veterans with mustard gas injury: 1919-1965. J. nat. Cancer Inst., 54, 311-317

Pierpont, H. & Davison, C. (1962) Lung perfusion. Behaviour of "alkylating" and "antimetabolite" cancer chemotherapeutic agents in dogs. J. Amer. med. Ass., 179, 421-423

Reid, B.D. & Walker, I.G. (1969) Response of mammalian cells to alkylating agents. II. On the mechanism of the removal of sulfur mustard-induced cross-links. Biochem. biophys. acta, 179, 179-188

Roberts, J.J. & Warwick, G.P. (1963) Studies of the mode of action of alkylating agents. VI. The metabolism of bis-2-chloroethylsulphide (mustard gas) and related compounds. Biochem. Pharmacol., 12, 1329-1334

Roberts, J.J., Brent, T.P. & Crathorn, A.R. (1971a) Evidence for the inactivation and repair of the mammalian DNA template after alkylation by mustard gas and half mustard gas. Europ. J. Cancer, 7, 515-524

Roberts, J.J., Pascoe, J.M., Smith, B.A. & Crathorn, A.R. (1971b) Quantitative aspects of the repair of alkylated DNA in cultured mammalian cells. II. Non-semiconservative DNA synthesis (repair synthesis) in HeLa and Chinese hamster cells following treatment with alkylating agents. Chem.-biol. Interact., 3, 49-68

Rose, S., ed. (1968) Chemical and Biological Warfare, Boston, Beacon Press, pp. 32-33

Rozmiarek, H., Capizzi, R.L., Papirmeister, B., Fuhrman, W.H. & Smith, W.J. (1973) Mutagenic activity in somatic and germ cells following chronic inhalation of sulfur mustard. Mutation Res., 21, 13-14

Scott, D., Fox, M. & Fox, B.W. (1974) The relationship between chromosomal aberrations, survival and DNA repair in tumour cell lines of differential sensitivity to X-rays and sulphur mustard. Mutation Res., 22, 207-221

Seidell, A. (1941) Solubilities of Organic Compounds, 3rd ed., Vol. II, New York, Van Nostrand Co. Inc., pp. 341-342

Stecher, P.G., ed. (1968) The Merck Index, 8th ed., Rahway, N.J., Merck & Co., p. 706

Thorpe, E., ed. (1974) Dictionary of Applied Chemistry, 4th ed., Vol. 3, London, Longman, p. 8

United Nations (1969) Chemical and Bacteriological (Biological) Weapons and the Effects of their Possible Use, New York, p. 2

Wada, S., Nishimoto, Y., Miyanishi, M., Kambe, S. & Miller, R.W. (1968) Mustard gas as a cause of respiratory neoplasia in man. Lancet, i, 1161-1163

Weiss, A. & Weiss, B. (1975) Karzinogenese durch Lost-Exposition beim Menschen, ein wichtiger Hinweis für die alkylantien-Therapie. Dtsch. med. Wschr., 100, 919-923

Yamada, A. (1963) On the late injuries following occupational inhalation of mustard gas, with special reference to carcinoma of the respiratory tract. Acta path. jap., 13, 131-155

Yamada, A., Hirose, F. & Miyanishi, M. (1953) An autopsy case of bronchial carcinoma found in a patient succumbed to occupational mustard gas poisoning. Gann, 44, 216-219

Yamada, A., Hirose, F., Nagai, M. & Nakamura, T. (1957) Five cases of cancer of the larynx found in persons who suffered from occupational mustard gas poisoning. Gann, 48, 366-368

1. Chemical and Physical Data

Nitrogen mustard

1.1 Synonyms and trade names

Chem. Abstr. Reg. Serial No.:   51-75-2

Chem. Abstr. Name: 2-Chloro-*N*-(2-chloroethyl)-*N*-methylethanamine

N,*N*'-Bis(2-chloroethyl)-*N*-methylamine; *N*,*N*-bis(2-chloroethyl)methyl-
amine; bis(2-chloroethyl)methylamine; bis(β-chloroethyl)methylamine;
chloramine*†; chlormethine; cloramin; β,β'-dichlorodiethyl-*N*-
methylamine; di(2-chloroethyl)methylamine; 2,2'-dichloro-*N*-methyl-
diethylamine; HN2*; MBA; mechlorethamine*; *N*-methyl-bis(2-chloro-
ethyl)amine; *N*-methyl-bis(β-chloroethyl)amine; methylbis(β-chloroethyl)amine; methylbis(chloroethylamine); *N*-methyl-2,2'-dichloro-
diethylamine; methyldi(2-chloroethyl)amine

Caryolysin*; Embichin*; Mustargen*; Mustine*; Mutagen*;
Nitrogen mustard*ψ

---

*This name is also used for the hydrochloride salt of nitrogen mustard.

†The term 'chloramine' or 'chloroamine' is used broadly to include all
compounds, both inorganic and organic, containing one or more chlorine
atoms attached to nitrogen. Specifically, 'chloramine' is used for the
compound NH_2Cl and for toluene-*para*-sulphonsodichloroamide trihydrate
(synonyms: Chloramine T, Chloraminum).

ψThis name has been used for other amines closely related to nitrogen
mustard, e.g., tris(2-chloroethyl)amine, $N(CH_2CH_2Cl)_3$, also known as HN3;
trichlormethine; 2,2'2"-trichlorotriethylamine; and tris(β-chloroethyl)-
amine.

1.2 Chemical formula and molecular weight

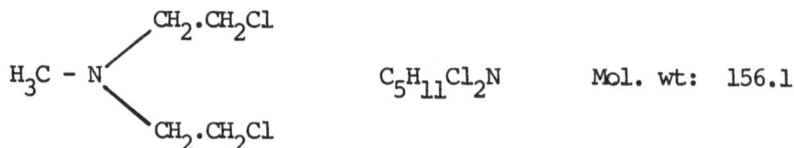

$$H_3C - N \begin{cases} CH_2.CH_2Cl \\ CH_2.CH_2Cl \end{cases}$$

$C_5H_{11}Cl_2N$ Mol. wt: 156.1

1.3 Chemical and physical properties of the pure substance

(a) Description: Liquid; faint fishy odour

(b) Melting-point: $-60^{\circ}C$

(c) Boiling-point: $87^{\circ}C$ at 18 mm Hg; $75^{\circ}C$ at 10 mm Hg; $64^{\circ}C$ at 5 mm Hg

(d) Density: d_4^{25} 1.118

(e) Identity test: Forms crystalline picrate (m.p., $132.7^{\circ}C$)

(f) Solubility: Very slightly soluble in water; miscible with dimethyl formamide, carbon disulphide, carbon tetrachloride and many other organic solvents and oils

(g) Volatility: Saturated air contains 3.6 mg/l at $25^{\circ}C$.

(h) Stability: Undiluted liquid decomposes slowly on standing and forms polymeric quaternary ammonium salts which are insoluble in the free base; reacts rapidly with water

1.4 Technical products and impurities

Nitrogen mustard (HN_2) is not produced commercially.

Nitrogen mustard hydrochloride

1.1 Synonyms and trade names

Chem. Abstr. Reg. Serial No.:   55-86-7

Chem. Abstr. Name: 2-Chloro-*N*-(2-chloroethyl)-*N*-methylethanamine hydrochloride

Azotoperite; *N,N*-bis(2-chloroethyl)methylamine hydrochloride;

bis(2-chloroethyl)methylamine hydrochloride; chloramin; chloramine*†; chlorethamine; chlorethazine; β,β'-dichlorodiethyl-*N*-methylamine hydrochloride; di(2-chloroethyl)methylamine hydrochloride; di(chloroethyl)methylamine hydrochloride; 2,2'-dichloro-*N*-methyl-diethylamine hydrochloride; dimitan; HN2*; HN2 hydrochloride; MBA hydrochloride; mechlorethamine*; mechlorethamine hydrochloride; *N*-methylbis(2-chloroethyl)amine hydrochloride; methylbis(2-chloroethyl)amine hydrochloride; *N*-methylbis(β-chloroethyl)amine hydrochloride; methylbis(β-chloroethyl)amine hydrochloride; *N*-methyl-2,2'-dichlorodiethylamine hydrochloride; methyldi(2-chloroethyl)amine hydrochloride; methyldi(β-chloroethyl)amine hydrochloride; N-Lost; NSC-762 hydrochloride

Caryolysine*; Dichloren; Embichin*; Embikhine; Erasol; Mebichloramine; Mitoxine; Mustargen*; Mustargen hydrochloride; Mustine*; Mustine Hydrochlor; Mustine hydrochloride; Mutagen*; Nitrogen mustard*; Nitrogranulogen

1.2 Chemical formula and molecular weight

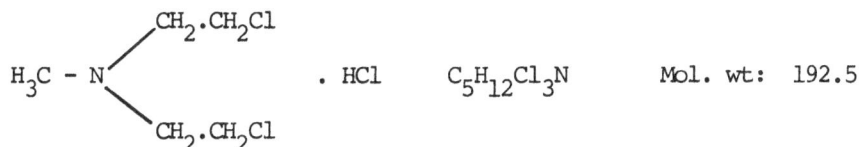

H₃C - N⟨CH₂.CH₂Cl / CH₂.CH₂Cl   . HCl $C_5H_{12}Cl_3N$ Mol. wt: 192.5

1.3 Chemical and physical properties of the pure substance

(a) Description: White, hygroscopic crystals

(b) Melting-point: 109-111°C

---

*This name is also used for nitrogen mustard; the word 'hydrochloride' is frequently omitted when the hydrochloride salt is meant.

†The term 'chloramine' or 'chloroamine' is used broadly to include all compounds, both inorganic and organic, containing one or more chlorine atoms attached to nitrogen. Specifically, 'chloramine' is used for the compound NH_2Cl and for toluene-*para*-sulphonsodichloroamide trihydrate (synonyms: Chloramine T, Chloraminum).

(c) **Identity test**: As given in the British Pharmacopoeia (British Pharmacopoeia Commission, 1973)

(d) **Solubility**: Soluble in water (1 g/100 ml) and in ethanol

(e) **Stability**: Dry crystals are stable; unstable in aqueous solution

1.4 Technical products and impurities

Nitrogen mustard (HN_2) hydrochloride is available in the US and Europe in powder form for intravenous injection. The powder is packaged in ampoules containing 3 or 10 mg of the active ingredient and 90 mg of sodium chloride, to be administered after solution in sterile water (Blacow, 1967; Calabresi & Parks, 1970; Dictionnaire Vidal, 1975; Pullom, 1968-69; Steinböck *et al.*, 1969). HN_2 hydrochloride for injection contains 100±10% of the labelled amount of active ingredient (US Pharmacopeial Convention, Inc., 1970), and the material used to formulate the injections contains 99±1.5% of the compound on an anhydrous basis.

2. Production, Use, Occurrence and Analysis

For important background information on this section, see preamble, p. 17.

Nitrogen mustard

2.1 Production and use

HN_2 can be prepared by treating *N*-methyldiethanolamine with thionyl chloride followed by treatment with caustic soda to release the free amine (Prelog & Stepan, 1935). It is not manufactured in commercial quantities in the US or Japan, and no evidence was found that this chemical is imported by either country. There is one producer in the UK (Chemical Information Services, Ltd, 1975).

HN_2 was produced in the past for use as a vesicant in chemical warfare. Although no military use was made of the chemical, stockpiles may have existed in the US as recently as 1974 (Anon., 1974).

It has been used as a chemical intermediate, e.g., the hydrochloride of the amine oxide produced from it is reported to be useful as an anti-

196

neoplastic agent, but no indication was found that this amine oxide is produced in the US. The only known commercial derivative of HN_2 is its hydrochloride, which has been used in limited quantities as an antineo-plastic agent.

Laboratory experiments have been conducted with HN_2 for use as a cross-linking agent in textiles (Roberts & Rowland, 1970; Rowland *et al.*, 1970). In the USSR it has been tested for use in sizing agents for cotton yarn, in grease for metal cutting, as a fungicide and as an antiviral aerosol disinfectant (Kremnev, 1971; Mandich, 1970; Osmanov, 1968; Slobodenyuk & Karpukhin, 1970).

2.2 Occurrence

HN_2 is not known to occur in nature.

Nitrogen mustard hydrochloride

2.1 Production and use

HN_2 hydrochloride can be prepared by treating *N*-methyldiethanolamine with thionyl chloride (Prelog & Stepan, 1935). It has been manufactured by one company in the US since 1950, and, according to industry sources, 1.5 kg of the chemical were manufactured and sold in 1974 in the US. HN_2 hydrochloride is also produced in the UK.

This chemical is used in human medicine as an antineoplastic agent, either alone, or in combination with other chemotherapeutic agents, in the treatment of neoplastic diseases, including Hodgkin's disease, leukaemia, generalized lymphosarcoma, mycosis fungoides and bronchogenic carcinoma. It is also used in controlling pleural, peritoneal or pericardial effusions due to metastatic tumours (Kastrup, 1974). The drug is administered by i.v. injection in a single total dose of 0.4 mg/kg bw or in 2 or 4 daily doses of 0.1-0.2 mg/kg bw (Merck *et al.*, 1974).

Clinical trials have been conducted to assess its usefulness as an immunosuppressant in the treatment of rheumatoid arthritis (McCarty & McLaughlin, 1968), in the treatment of a variety of other non-malignant diseases (Skinner & Schwartz, 1972) and in tissue transplantation studies (Russell & Monaco, 1964).

197

In veterinary medicine HN_2 hydrochloride is reported to be used for the treatment of lymphosarcoma and of mast-cell sarcoma in dogs and of fowl leukosis (Stecher, 1968).

Its use as a chemosterilant (Flint *et al.*, 1968; LaChance *et al.*, 1969) and as a cross-linking agent in the manufacture of ion-exchange fibres (Rulison, 1968) have also been investigated.

2.2 Occurrence

HN_2 hydrochloride is not known to occur in nature.

Nitrogen mustard and nitrogen mustard hydrochloride

2.3 Analysis

Free HN_2 or its hydrochloride can be determined colorimetrically by reaction with 4-(4'-nitrobenzyl)pyridine (Friedman & Boger, 1961; Obrecht *et al.*, 1964; Tan & Cole, 1965; Truhaut *et al.*, 1963). Determinations of HN_2 hydrochloride have been made using paper and thin-layer chromatographic methods (Sakurai & Ito, 1960; Walthier & Jeney, 1968); a fluorometric method for its determination in biological materials, with a sensitivity of 0.02 µg/ml (Mellet & Woods, 1960), and titrimetric methods (British Pharmacopoeia Commission, 1973) have also been described.

3. Biological Data Relevant to the Evaluation of Carcinogenic Risk to Man

3.1 Carcinogenicity and related studies in animals

(a) Skin application

Mouse: Skin application of HN2 hydrochloride in water to "white" mice did not induce skin tumours (Narpozzi, 1953).

(b) Subcutaneous and/or intramuscular administration

Mouse: A group of 20 stock mice was given weekly s.c. injections of 1 mg/kg bw HN2 hydrochloride for 50 weeks. Of a total of 10 mice surviving 284-580 days, 6 had tumours: 3 lung carcinomas, 1 lung adenoma, 1 lymphosarcoma in the liver and 1 uterine fibromyoma. Tumours (6 lung adenomas and 2 hepatomas) occurred in 8/40 untreated controls killed between 420-540 days of age (Boyland & Horning, 1949). [P<0.05].

Tumours at the site of injection (sarcomas, skin papillomas and squamous-cell carcinomas) developed in 3/15 C3H mice of both sexes, in 5/21 male C3H mice and in 3/37 male C3Hf mice given 8 weekly s.c. injections of 0.025 mg HN2 hydrochloride in water. No skin tumours appeared in 14 C3H mice of both sexes, in 21 male C3H or in 39 male C3Hf non-treated control mice (P<0.001). The incidences of pulmonary tumours in test groups *versus* those in control groups were 5/15 *versus* 3/14 for C3H mice of both sexes, 8/21 *versus* 5/21 for male C3H mice and 21/37 *versus* 6/39 for male C3Hf mice. The 47% incidence of pulmonary tumours in treated mice was significantly greater than the 19% incidence in the combined controls (P<0.001). No difference between test and control mice was seen in respect of other remote tumours (Heston, 1953).

(c) Intraperitoneal administration

Mouse: Four groups of 60 A/J mice of both sexes, 4-6 weeks old, received 12 i.p. injections of HN2 hydrochloride in water during 4 weeks (total doses, 3.85, 212, 866 and 3369 µg/kg bw). The numbers of mice surviving the 39 weeks of the experiment were 47, 53, 51 and 38 in the four groups; a dose-related increase in the number of lung tumours was observed. The incidences of lung tumours in the four groups were 30%, 40%, 69% and 95%, with 0.3, 0.6, 1.2 and 2.8 lung tumours per mouse. A smaller increase in the number of lung tumours was seen in four groups of 30 A/J mice given total doses by i.p. injection in tricaprylin of 46, 206, 828 and 3311 µg/ kg bw HN2 hydrochloride. The numbers of mice surviving 39 weeks were 26, 28, 28 and 30, and 46%, 50%, 29% and 63% developed lung tumours, with 0.8, 0.6, 0.4 and 1.0 lung tumours per mouse. The lung tumour incidences were 37% (0.48 tumours/mouse) and 27% (0.29) in 157 male and 182 female control mice given 12 i.p. injections of water and 36% (0.47) and 32% (0.42) in 55 male and 53 female control mice given a similar number of injections of tricaprylin alone and killed at 39 weeks. An increased incidence of tumours at other sites was not apparent. In the same experiment the potency of HN2 hydrochloride was reported to be about one-third that of uracil mustard on a molar basis (Shimkin *et al.*, 1966). This study confirms previous results obtained by Duhig (1965).

(d) Intravenous administration

Mouse: A group of 37 male and female A mice, 2-3 months old, received
2-4 i.v. injections of 1 mg/kg bw HN2 hydrochloride in 0.01 ml distilled
water at 2-day intervals; 38 controls received distilled water alone.
After 16 weeks, 29/29 test mice examined had developed lung tumours (3.5
tumours/mouse), compared with 4/30 controls (0.17 tumours/mouse) (Heston,
1949).

Further work by Heston (1950) revealed a lung tumour incidence of 100%
(9.6 tumours/mouse) in another group of 20 A mice which received 4 similar
injections of HN2 hydrochloride (total dose, 0.1 mg) and were allowed to
live for 10 months; the incidence was 62% in 32 controls (0.81 tumours/
mouse). After a single injection of 0.4 mg/kg bw HN2 hydrochloride, all 9
survivors at 10 months showed lung tumours (7.5 tumours/mouse); lung
tumours occurred in 18/31 controls (0.94 tumours/mouse).

In 104 female RF mice, 10 weeks old, injected intravenously with 4
doses of 2.4 mg/kg bw HN2 as a 0.1% solution in saline at 2-week intervals,
with observation up to 2 years, increased incidences of thymic lymphomas
(21% *versus* 10% in 112 controls [P<0.05]) and pulmonary adenomas (68% *versus*
15% in controls [P<0.001]) were observed. The average ages at death were
490 days in treated mice and 632 days in controls (Conklin *et al.*, 1965).

Rat: A group of 48 male BR46 rats, 100 days old, received 52 weekly
i.v. injections of 0.11 mg/kg bw HN2 hydrochloride (total dose, 5.72 mg/
kg bw). Of the rats surviving at the appearance of the first tumour, 7/27
(26%) developed malignant tumours and 5/27 (18%) developed benign tumours,
compared with 4/65 (6%) and 3/65 (5%) controls. The average observation
time of the tumours was 16 months in treated rats and 23 months in controls.
The malignant tumours occurring in treated rats were 1 lymphatic and 1
myeloid leukaemia, 1 reticulum-cell sarcoma, 1 liposarcoma, 1 adenocarcinoma
of the large intestine, 1 sarcoma of the meninges and 1 haemangioendothelioma of the salivary gland. In controls 3 mammary sarcomas and 1 malignant
phaechromocytoma, 2 thymomas and 1 mammary fibroma were observed (Schmähl
& Osswald, 1970). [P<0.05].

(e) Other experimental systems

Foetal lung tissue from BALB/c _mice_ was exposed to HN2 hydrochloride at concentrations of $1:5 \times 10^4 - 1:5 \times 10^6$ Ringer's solution for 15-60 minutes and then implanted as a suspension into the thigh muscles of young adult mice of the same strain. The implants were examined 10 weeks to 6 months later and some were found to contain typical pulmonary adenomas. No adenomas appeared in lung tissue implants not previously exposed to HN2 hydrochloride (Rogers, 1955).

3.2 Other relevant biological data

The LD_{50} of HN2 in mice and rats by s.c. and i.v. injection is about 1-4 mg/kg bw. The oral LD_{50} in mice is 10-20 mg/kg bw, depending upon whether the animals receive food prior to dosing or not (Anslow _et al._, 1947; Boyland, 1946). The i.v. LD_{50} of HN2 hydrochloride in rats is 1.1 mg/kg bw (Stecher, 1968).

An i.v. dose of 3 mg/kg bw HN2 administered to dogs rapidly disappeared from the blood: 0.01% was found in the urine, and low levels were found in the tissues, the highest concentration being in the bone marrow. A 90% breakdown of HN2 occurred within 4 minutes of incubation with whole blood (Mellet & Woods, 1960). Ishidate (1959) also demonstrated the almost immediate disappearance of $^{14}CH_3$-labelled HN2 from the blood of dogs given 0.5 mg/kg intravenously over 5 seconds or 60 minutes, and a low urinary excretion of HN2. Mice given 35 mg/kg bw HN2 hydrochloride intravenously and examined by autoradiography had significant levels of the compound in brain, spinal cord, lungs and submaxillary glands (Tubaro & Bulgini, 1968). In rats, 16% of an injected dose of HN2 was found present in the spleen, lungs, kidneys, liver and blood, and 17% was excreted in the urine (Obrecht _et al._, 1964).

Following its _in vivo_ administration, HN2 or its hydrochloride is probably converted into an ethyleneimmonium ion which reacts with the guanine residues in adjacent strands of DNA as well as with SH groups (Boyland, 1946; Verly, 1964).

HN2 is embryotoxic in rats when given by i.v. injection on the 4th day of pregnancy (Brock & Kreybig, 1964); it also causes foetal abnormalities in rats (Murphy *et al.*, 1958). When injected intradermally into coloured mice, HN2 causes local greying of hair (Boyland & Sargent, 1951).

HN2 induces point mutations in *Escherichia coli* B/M12 (Bryson, 1948) and in conidia of strain 5256A of *Neurospora crassa* (McElroy *et al.*, 1947) and causes chromosome aberrations in a variety of plants and mammals (see Loveless, 1966). Inductions by HN2 of dominant lethal mutations in ICR/Ha Swiss mice (Epstein *et al.*, 1972) and of IUdR-resistant variants in P388 mouse lymphoma cells (Anderson & Fox, 1974) have been reported.

HN2 hydrochloride produces the same mutagenic effects as HN2: it induces reverse mutations in *Aspergillus nidulans* (Kovalenko *et al.*, 1969) and in *Escherichia coli* Sd-4-73 (Iyer & Szybalski, 1958) and visible recessive mutations and inherited semi-sterility in CBA mice (Falconer *et al.*, 1952).

Sokal & Lessmann (1960) reported on four women with Hodgkin's disease who were treated with HN2 during the first and third (1 case) or second and third (3 cases) trimesters of pregnancy. No abnormalities were recorded in the offspring at 2 months, $8\frac{1}{2}$, $7\frac{1}{2}$ and $9\frac{1}{2}$ years.

3.3 Observations in man

No data were available to the Working Group. However, see also mustard gas, p. 181.

4. Comments on Data Reported and Evaluation[1]

4.1 Animal data

Nitrogen mustard, administered mainly as the hydrochloride, is carcinogenic in mice and rats. Following its subcutaneous, intraperitoneal or intravenous injection, it produced an increased incidence of lung tumours and thymic lymphomas in mice; it produced a variety of malignant tumours in rats following its intravenous injection.

---

[1]See also the section, "Animal Data in Relation to the Evaluation of Risk to Man" in the introduction to this volume, p. 15.

4.2 Human data

No case reports or epidemiological studies referring to exposures to nitrogen mustard alone were available to the Working Group.

5. References

Anderson, D. & Fox, M. (1974) The induction of thymidine- and IUdR-resistant variants in P388 mouse lymphoma cells by X-rays, UV and mono- and bifunctional alkylating agents. Mutation Res., 25, 107-122

Anon. (1974) House stirs up chemical warfare issue. Chemical and Engineering News, August 19, pp. 19-20

Anslow, W.P., Jr, Karnovsky, D.A., Val Jager, B. & Smith, H.W. (1947) The toxicity and pharmacological action of the nitrogen mustards and certain related compounds. J. Pharmacol. exp. Ther., 91, 224-235

Blacow, N.W., ed. (1967) Martindale: The Extra Pharmacopoeia, London, The Pharmaceutical Press

Boyland, E. (1946) The toxicity of alkyl-bis-(β-chloroethyl)-amines and of the products of their reaction with water. Brit. J. Pharmacol., 1, 247-254

Boyland, E. & Horning, E.S. (1949) The induction of tumours with nitrogen mustards. Brit. J. Cancer, 3, 118-123

Boyland, E. & Sargent, S. (1951) The local greying of hair in mice treated with X-rays and radiomimetic drugs. Brit. J. Cancer, 5, 433-440

British Pharmacopoeia Commission (1973) British Pharmacopoeia, London, HMSO, p. 311

Brock, N. & Kreybig, Th.V. (1964) Determination of the teratogenic effect of pharmaceuticals on rats. Arch. exp. Path. Pharmacol., 249, 117-145

Bryson, V. (1948) The effects of nitrogen mustard on *Escherichia coli*. J. Bact., 56, 423-433

Calabresi, P. & Parks, R.E., Jr (1970) Alkylating agents, antimetabolites, hormones and other antiproliferative agents. In: Goodman, L.S. & Gilman, A., eds, The Pharmacological Basis of Therapeutics, 4th ed., London, MacMillan, p. 1354

Chemical Information Services, Ltd (1975) Directory of Western European Chemical Producers, 1975/76, Oceanside, NY

Conklin, J.W., Upton, A.C. & Christenberry, K.W. (1965) Further observations on late somatic effects of radiomimetic chemicals and X-rays in mice. Cancer Res., 25, 20-28

Dictionnaire Vidal (1975) 51st ed., Paris, Office de Vulgarisation Pharmaceutique, p. 278

Duhig, J.T. (1965) Tumor incidence in A strain mice. Arch. Path., 79, 177-184

Epstein, S.S., Arnold, E., Andrea, J., Bass, W. & Bishop, Y. (1972) Detection of chemical mutagens by the dominant lethal assay in the mouse. Toxicol. appl. Pharmacol., 23, 288-325

Falconer, D.S., Slizynski, B.M. & Auerbach, C. (1952) Genetical effects of nitrogen mustard in the house mouse. J. Genet., 51, 81-88

Flint, H.M., Klassen, W., Norland, J. & Kressin, E. (1968) Chemosterilization of the tobacco budworm: survey of 16 compounds fed to adult moths. J. econ. Entomol., 61, 1726-1729

Friedman, O.M. & Boger, E. (1961) Colorimetric estimation of nitrogen mustards in aqueous media. Hydrolytic behavior of bis(beta-chloroethyl)amine or HN2. Analyt. Chem., 33, 906-910

Heston, W.E. (1949) Induction of pulmonary tumors in strain A mice with methylbis(β-chloroethyl)amine hydrochloride. J. nat. Cancer Inst., 10, 125-130

Heston, W.E. (1950) Carcinogenic action of the mustards. J. nat. Cancer Inst., 11, 415-423

Heston, W.E. (1953) Occurrence of tumors in mice injected subcutaneously with sulphur mustard and nitrogen mustard. J. nat. Cancer Inst., 14, 131-140

Ishidate, M. (1959) The mode of action of nitrogen mustard N-oxide. Acta Un. int. Cancr, 15, 139-144

Iyer, V.N. & Szybalski, W. (1958) Two simple methods for the detection of chemical mutagens. Appl. Microbiol., 6, 23-29

Kastrup, E.K., ed. (1974) Facts and Comparisons, St Louis, Missouri, Facts & Comparisons, Inc.

Kovalenko, S.P., Vovrish, P.E. & Panchenko, V.K. (1969) Mutagenic activity of some nitrogen mustards on *Aspergillus nidulans*. Tsitol. i Genet., 3, 252-254

Kremnev, M.G. (1971) Poly(vinyl alcohol) sizing composition for cotton yarn. Tekst. Prom. (Moscow), 31, 36-37

LaChance, L.E., Degrugillier, M. & Leverich, A.P. (1969) Comparative effects of chemosterilants on spermatogenic stages in the housefly. I. Induction of dominant lethal mutations in mature sperm and gonial cell death. Mutation Res., 7, 63-74

Loveless, A. (1966) Genetic and Allied Effects of Alkylating Agents, London, Butterworth

Mandich, F.I. (1970) USSR Patent, 282,568, September 28, Ukranian Printing Institute

McCarty, D.L., Jr & McLaughlin, G. (1968) Clinical uses of anti-inflammatory drugs. In: Rabinowitz, J.L. & Myerson, R.M., eds, Topics in Medicinal Chemistry, Vol. 2, New York, Interscience, pp. 217-246

McElroy, W.D., Cushing, J.E. & Miller, H. (1947) The induction of biochemical mutations in *Neurospora crassa* by nitrogen mustard. J. Cell comp. Physiol., 30, 331-346

Mellet, L.B. & Woods, L.A. (1960) The fluorometric estimation of mechlorethamine (mustargen) and its biological disposition in the dog. Cancer Res., 20, 518-523

Merck, Sharp & Dohme (1974) Direction Circular: Trituration of Mustargen (Mechlorethamine HCl for Injection, MSD), March, West Point, Pennsylvania, Merck & Co. Inc.

Murphy, M.L., Del Moro, A. & Lacon, C. (1958) The comparative effects of five polyfunctional alkylating agents on the rat fetus, with additional notes on the chick embryo. Ann. N.Y. Acad. Sci., 68, 762-782

Narpozzi, A. (1953) Sull' azione cancerigena dell' azoiprite. Riv. Anat. pat., 6, 1155-1170

Obrecht, P., Woenkhaus, J.W. & Strickstrock, K.H. (1964) Zum Nachweis von N-Methyl-bis-chloräthylamin (Dichloren) im Organismus der Ratte durch 4-*p*-Nitrobenzyl-pyridin (NPB). Z. Krebsforsch., 66, 151-154

Osmanov, S.I. (1968) Comparative study of the fungicidal capacity of chemical substances for *Aspergillus, Penicillium* and *Trichophyton* fungi. Sb. Nauch. Rab. Dagestan. Nauch.-Issled. Vet. Inst., 2, 91-92

Prelog, V. & Stepan, V. (1935) Bis(β-haloethyl)amines. VII. A new synthesis of N-monoalkylpiperazines. Coll. Czech. chem. Commun., 7, 93-102

Pullom, E.N., ed. (1968-69) Mims Annual Compendium, London, Medical Publications Ltd, p. 85

Roberts, E.J. & Rowland, S.P. (1970) Synthesis of the substituted and crosslinked glucoses corresponding to the structural units in a cotton cellulose modified with N-methylbis(2-chloroethyl)amine. Canad. J. Chem., 48, 1383-1390

Rogers, S. (1955) The *in vitro* initiation of pulmonary adenomas in mouse lung tissue with nitrogen mustard. I. The influences of concentration of agent, duration of exposure and mitotic state of the tissue at the time of exposure. J. nat. Cancer Inst., 15, 1379-1390

Rowland, S.P., Roberts, E.J. & Brannan, M.A.F. (1970) Relating wrinkle recovery to the structure of reagent residues in crosslinked cottons. Text. Chem. Color., 2, 373-377

Rulison, R.N. (1968) Ion-exchange fibers. US Patent, 3,379,719, April 23, Celanese Corp.

Russell, P.S. & Monaco, A.P. (1964) The biology of tissue transplantation. New Engl. J. Med., 271, 664-671

Sakurai, Y. & Ito, K. (1960) Paper chromatographic detection of nitrogen mustard. Chem. pharm. Bull., 8, 655-656

Schmähl, D. & Osswald, H. (1970) Experimentelle Untersuchungen über carcinogene Wirkungen von Krebs-Chemotherapeutica und Immunosuppressiva. Arzneimittel-Forsch., 20, 1461-1467

Shimkin, M.B., Weisburger, J.H., Weisburger, E.K., Gubareff, N. & Suntzeff, V. (1966) Bioassay of 29 alkylating chemicals by the pulmonary-tumor response in strain A mice. J. nat. Cancer Inst., 36, 915-935

Skinner, M.D. & Schwartz, R.S. (1972) Immunosuppressive therapy. New Engl. J. Med., 287, 221-227, 281-286

Slobodenyuk, V.K. & Karpukhin, G.I. (1970) Experimental substantiation of the aerosol method of disinfection in viral infections. II. Inactivating action of hydrogen peroxide, chloramine and hexylresorcinol aerosols on various viruses in the air and on surfaces. Zh. Mikrobiol. (Moscow), 47, 113-117

Sokal, J.E. & Lessmann, E.M. (1960) Effects of cancer therapeutic agents on the human foetus. J. Amer. med. Ass., 172, 1765-1771

Stecher, P.G., ed. (1968) The Merck Index, 8th ed., Rahway, N.J., Merck & Co., pp. 646-647

Steinböck, R., Zekert, F. & Zimmermann, G. (1969) Austria-Codex: 1969/1970, Vienna, Österreichischer Apotheker-Verlag, p. 480

Tan, Y.L. & Cole, D.R. (1965) New method for determination of alkylating agents in biologic fluids. Clin. Chem., 11, 58-62

Truhaut, R., Delacoux, E., Brule, G. & Bohuon, C. (1963) Dosage des agents alcoylants dans les milieux biologiques. Méthode utilisant la réaction colorée avec la γ-(nitro-4-benzyl)-pyridine en milieu alcalin. Clin. chim. acta, 8, 235-245

Tubaro, E. & Bulgini, M.J. (1968) Cytotoxic and antifungal agents: their body distribution and tissue affinity. Nature (Lond.), 218, 395-396

US Pharmacopeial Convention, Inc. (1970) The US Pharmacopeia, 18th rev., Easton, Pa , Mack, pp. 383-384

Verly, W.G. (1964) Action mutagène et cancérigène des agents alcoylants. Rev. franç. Etud. clin. biol., 9, 878-883

Walthier, J. & Jeney, A., Jr (1968) Biologiai alkilezo agensek réteg-kromatografiaja. Acta pharm. hung., 38, 236-244

NITROGEN MUSTARD N-OXIDE (HYDROCHLORIDE)

1. Chemical and Physical Data

Nitrogen mustard N-oxide

1.1 Synonyms and trade names

Chem. Abstr. Reg. Serial No.: 126-85-2

Chem. Abstr. Name: 2-Chloro-*N*-(2-chloroethyl)-*N*-methylethanamine-*N*-oxide

2,2'-Dichloro-*N*-methyldiethylamine-*N*-oxide; HN2 oxide mustard; MBAO; mechlorethamine oxide; methylbis(β-chloroethyl)amine-*N*-oxide; nitrogen mustard amine oxide; nitrogen mustard oxide*; nitrogen mustard *N*-oxide*; NMO; oxy-NH2

1.2 Chemical formula and molecular weight

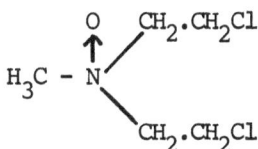

$$H_3C - N \begin{matrix} \uparrow O \\ \diagup \ CH_2.CH_2Cl \\ \diagdown \ CH_2.CH_2Cl \end{matrix}$$

C₅H₁₁Cl₂NO   Mol. wt: 172

$C_5H_{11}Cl_2NO$ Mol. wt: 172

1.3 Chemical and physical properties of the pure substance

(a) Solubility: Soluble in water; sparingly soluble in benzene and ether

(b) Stability: In the presence of heavy metal ions it may decompose to formaldehyde and secondary amines. In alkaline solutions (pH 8) it decomposes rapidly, with liberation of chloride.

1.4 Technical products and impurities

Nitrogen mustard (HN2) *N*-oxide is not produced commercially.

---

*This name is frequently used when the hydrochloride salt is meant.

Nitrogen mustard N-oxide hydrochloride

1.1 Synonyms and trade names

Chem. Abstr. Reg. Serial No.: 302-70-5

Chem. Abstr. Name: 2-Chloro-*N*-(2-chloroethyl)-*N*-methylethanamine-*N*-oxide hydrochloride

2,2'-Dichloro-*N*-methyldiethylamine *N*-oxide hydrochloride; mechlor-ethamine oxide hydrochloride; methylbis(2-chloroethyl)amine *N*-oxide hydrochloride; methylbis(β-chloroethyl)amine *N*-oxide hydrochloride; *N*-methylbis(β-chloroethyl)amine *N*-oxide hydrochloride; *N*-methyl-2,2'-dichlorodiethylamine *N*-oxide hydrochloride; methyldi(2-chloro-ethyl)amine *N*-oxide hydrochloride; nitrogen mustard oxide*; nitrogen mustard *N*-oxide*; nitrogen mustard *N*-oxide hydrochloride; N-Oxyd-Lost; NSC-10107; SK-598

Mitomen; Mustron; Nitromin; Nitromin hydrochloride

1.2 Chemical formula and molecular weight

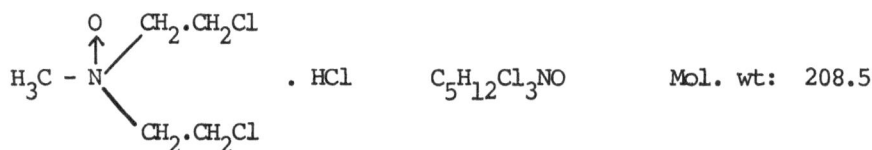

$$H_3C - N \overset{\overset{O}{\uparrow}}{\underset{CH_2.CH_2Cl}{\overset{CH_2.CH_2Cl}{\diagup}}} \quad . HCl \qquad C_5H_{12}Cl_3NO \qquad Mol. \; wt: \; 208.5$$

1.3 Chemical and physical properties of the pure substance

(a) Description: Colourless, odourless crystals

(b) Melting-point: 109-110°C

(c) Solubility: Freely soluble in water and ethanol; slightly soluble in benzene and ether

(d) Stability: Hydrolyses in alkaline solution (pH 8), much more slowly than does the free base

---

*This name is also used for the free base.

<u>(e) Reactivity</u>: Forms picrate (m.p., 122-124°C); readily reduced, e.g., releases iodine from potassium iodide

1.4 Technical products and impurities

Nitrogen mustard (HN2) *N*-oxide hydrochloride is available in Austria and Japan in the form of tablets containing 5 mg active ingredient and in ampoules for intravenous injection containing 25 and 50 mg (JAPTA, 1973; Steinböck *et al.*, 1969).

2. Production, Use, Occurrence and Analysis

For important background information on this section, see preamble, p. 17.

Nitrogen mustard *N*-oxide

2.1 Production and use

HN2 *N*-oxide can be prepared by treating 2,2'-dichloro-*N*-methyldiethyl-amine with hydrogen peroxide and acetic anhydride (Sakurai & Izumi, 1953). Although it is believed to have been tested experimentally as an anti-neoplastic agent, this chemical is not manufactured or imported in commercial quantities in the US or Europe.

The only commercial use for HN2 *N*-oxide is believed to be as a chemical intermediate in the manufacture of HN2 *N*-oxide hydrochloride, which is marketed in Europe and Japan as an antineoplastic agent (JAPTA, 1973; Steinböck *et al.*, 1969).

2.2 Occurrence

HN2 *N*-oxide is not known to occur in nature.

Nitrogen mustard *N*-oxide hydrochloride

2.1 Production and use

HN2 *N*-oxide hydrochloride can be prepared by treating 2,2'-dichloro-*N*-methyldiethylamine with hydrogen peroxide and acetic anhydride followed by hydrochloric acid (Aiko *et al.*, 1952).

In the US, HN2 *N*-oxide hydrochloride has never been produced or marketed as a commercial product; however, it has been tested for use as an antineoplastic agent (Bratzel *et al.*, 1963) and as an insect chemosterilant (Crystal, 1963; Gouck & LaBrecque, 1964). This chemical was produced in the Federal Republic of Germany and was used as an antineoplastic agent to be administered intravenously (Steinböck *et al.*, 1969).

In Japan HN2 *N*-oxide hydrochloride has been used in human medicine as an antineoplastic agent for the treatment of lymphomas and oat-cell carcinomas of the lung. It is administered orally in doses of 0.5 mg/kg bw daily for 5-12 days or intravenously in doses of 0.5-2 mg/kg bw daily (Brulé *et al.*, 1973; JAPTA, 1973). Studies on the immunosuppressive effects of this chemical in the treatment of such diseases as nephrotic syndrome and in skin grafting have been made in that country (Nakao & Umetsu, 1967; Shimizu, 1971).

2.2 Occurrence

HN2 *N*-oxide hydrochloride is not known to occur in nature.

2.3 Analysis

Large amounts (2-10 mg) of HN2 *N*-oxide hydrochloride can be determined using titrimetric methods after reaction with potassium iodide; smaller amounts (0.01-0.06 mg) were measured colorimetrically after reaction with potassium iodide (Said *et al.*, 1961). A chromatographic separation technique has been described (Aiko *et al.*, 1952).

3. Biological Data Relevant to the Evaluation of Carcinogenic Risk to Man

3.1 Carcinogenicity and related studies in animals

(a) Skin application

Mouse: Three groups, 6 female C3H/He mice, 13 Al mice of both sexes and 25 ddCF2 mice of both sexes, 8-10 weeks of age, were given daily skin applications of 0.05 ml of a 1% solution of HN2 *N*-oxide (probably as the hydrochloride) in acetone on 6 days per week for 17-20 weeks. Of 37 mice surviving longer than 21 weeks, 9 developed tumours between 33-74 weeks after the start of the experiment. No tumours were found in a total of 46 control mice surviving longer than 21 weeks (Matsuyama *et al.*, 1966).

[Since the maximum survival of controls was not reported and the numbers of both control and treated animals are small, this study cannot be evaluated.]

(b) Subcutaneous and/or intramuscular administration

Mouse: Four weekly s.c. doses of 650 mg/kg bw (50% of the minimum lethal dose) of a 3% solution of HN2 N-oxide hydrochloride in saline were given to male and female dd/I suckling mice, 7 days old. Thymic lymphomas were observed in 27/47 and lung adenomas in 20/47 treated mice surviving 80 or more days. Lung carcinomas and Harderian gland adenomas also occurred in 8/38 and 6/38 mice surviving after 180 days. Other tumours occurring in treated mice, but not in saline-treated controls, that survived 180 or more days included 2 liver tumours, 2 ovarian tumours, 1 haemangioma of the duodenum and 1 forestomach papilloma. In 69 saline-treated controls surviving 80-450 days, 15 mice died with lung adenomas. The average survival time in treated mice was 260 days (Matsuyama et al., 1969).

(c) Intravenous administration

Rat: A group of 55 male BR46 rats, 60-70 days old, received weekly i.v. injections of 4.2 mg/kg bw HN2 N-oxide hydrochloride for 52 weeks (total dose, 218 mg/kg bw). Of 44 rats surviving at the appearance of the first tumour, 12 (27%) developed malignant tumours and 2 (4%), benign tumours, compared with 4/65 (6%) and 3/65 (5%) controls, respectively. The average observation time of the tumours was 16 months in treated animals and 23 months in controls. In treated rats, 3 sarcomas in the abdominal cavity, 7 reticular-cell tumours, 1 osteosarcoma and 1 angiosarcoma in the muscle were observed. Malignant tumours in controls included 3 mammary sarcomas and 1 phaeochromocytoma (Schmähl & Osswald, 1970). [P<0.01].

(d) Other experimental systems

Three groups, 51 dt mice, 47 ddN mice and 29 ddN mice, received twice weekly injections of 5 or 10 mg/kg bw or weekly injections of 20 mg/kg bw HN2 N-oxide hydrochloride in saline for 15 weeks, respectively. The injections were given by the i.p., i.v. or s.c. route in all groups. Twenty ddN mice served as controls and were not injected. The numbers of tumours occurring in treated animals surviving 26-80 weeks within each group were 15/21 (71%), 9/28 (32%) and 4/16 (25%), compared with 0/16 controls. Tumours in treated animals were mainly lymphomas, fibrosarcomas and pulmonary adenomas; 1 haemangioma of the liver and 1 adenoma of the parathyroid gland were also observed (Tokuoka, 1960).

3.2 Other relevant biological data

The i.v. LD$_{50}$ in rats is 60 mg/kg bw (Schmähl & Osswald, 1970).

After i.v. injection of 5 mg/kg bw ^{14}C-CH$_3$-HN2 N-oxide in dogs, virtually no activity was found in the blood after one hour. In the urine, the highest level of radioactivity was found between 5 and 20 minutes after the injection and had declined to zero after 4 hours (Ishidate, 1959).

HN2 N-oxide hydrochloride induces chromatid aberrations in Ehrlich-ascites tumour cells grown in mouse peritoneum (Rieger et al., 1969), point mutations in bacteria (Iyer & Szybalski, 1958; Szybalski, 1958) and dominant lethal mutations in mice (Ehling, 1974).

3.3 Observations in man

No data were available to the Working Group.

4. Comments on Data Reported and Evaluation[1]

4.1 Animal data

Nitrogen mustard N-oxide hydrochloride is carcinogenic in mice and rats. Following its subcutaneous injection in mice, it produced lung tumours, thymic lymphomas and Harderian gland adenomas; following its intravenous injection in rats it produced mainly lymphoreticular tumours and sarcomas.

4.2 Human data

No case reports or epidemiological studies were available to the Working Group.

---

[1]See also the section, "Animal Data in Relation to the Evaluation of Risk to Man" in the introduction to this volume, p. 15.

5. References

Aiko, I., Owari, S. & Torigoe, M. (1952) Nitrogen mustard *N*-oxide and its effect on the Yoshida sarcoma. J. pharm. Soc. Japan, 72, 1297-1300

Bratzel, R.P., Ross, R.B., Goodridge, T.H., Huntress, W.T., Flather, M.T. & Johnson, D.E. (1963) Survey of nitrogen mustards. Cancer Chemother. Rep., 26, 1-322

Brulé, G., Eckhardt, S.J., Hall, T.C. & Winkler, A. (1973) Drug Therapy of Cancer, Geneva, World Health Organization, p. 43

Crystal, M.M. (1963) The induction of sexual sterility in the screwworm fly by antimetabolites and alkylating agents. J. econ. Entomol., 56, 468-473

Ehling, U.H. (1974) Differential spermatogenic response of mice to the induction of mutations by antineoplastic drugs. Mutation Res., 26, 285-295

Gouck, H.K. & LaBrecque, G.C. (1964) Chemicals affecting fertility in adult houseflies. J. econ. Entomol., 57, 663-664

Ishidate, M. (1959) The mode of action of nitrogen mustard *N*-oxide. Acta Un. int. Cancr., 15, 139-144

Iyer, V.N. & Szybalski, W. (1958) Two simple methods for the detection of chemical mutagens. Appl. Microbiol., 6, 23-29

JAPTA (Japan Pharmaceutical Traders' Association) (1973) Japanese Drug Directory, Tokyo, p. 505

Matsuyama, M., Maekawa, A. & Nakamura, T. (1966) Biological studies of anticancer agents. II. Effect of percutaneous application. Gann, 57, 295-298

Matsuyama, M., Suzuki, H. & Nakamura, T. (1969) Carcinogenesis in dd/I mice injected during suckling period with urethane, nitrogen mustard *N*-oxide and nitroso-urethane. Brit. J. Cancer, 23, 167-171

Nakao, T. & Umetsu, M. (1967) Immunosuppressive treatment in steroid-resistant nephrotic syndrome. J. clin. Paediat., 15, 153-158

Rieger, R., Michaelis, A., Schöneich, J., Fischer, G.W. & Lohs, Kh. (1969) Über die Induktion von Chromatidenaberrationen durch quartäre *N*-Acylvinyl-Stickstofflost-Verbindungen. Stud. biophys., 17, 205-212

Said, E.F., Amer, M.M. & Said, A.A. (1961) Estimation of nitromin. Congr. Sci. Farm. Conf. Comun. Pisa, 21, 475-479

Sakurai, Y. & Izumi, M. (1953) N-Oxides of β-chloroethylamine derivatives. Pharm. Bull. (Tokyo), 1, 297-301

Schmähl, D. & Osswald, H. (1970) Experimentelle Untersuchungen über carcinogene Wirkungen von Krebs-Chemotherapeutica und Immunosuppressiva. Arzneimittel-Forsch., 20, 1461-1467

Shimizu, H. (1971) Studies on the screening of antitumor agents inhibiting the immune response and drug-induced chimera with cyclophosphamide. J. Nara med. Ass., 22, 305-323

Steinböck, R., Zekert, F. & Zimmermann, G. (1969) Austria-Codex: 1969/70, Vienna, Osterreichischer Apotheker-Verlag, p. 487

Szybalski, W. (1958) Special microbiological systems. II. Observations on chemical mutagenesis in microorganisms. Ann. N.Y. Acad. Sci., 76, 475-489

Tokuoka, S. (1960) Patho-anatomical studies on mice treated with nitrogen mustard N-oxide. Hiroshima J. med. Sci., 8, 479-518

1.   Chemical and Physical Data

1.1   Synonyms and trade names

Chem. Abstr. Reg. Serial No.: 22966-79-6

Chem. Abstr. Name: Estra-1,3,5(10)-triene-3,17β-diol,bis({*para*-[bis-
(2-chloroethyl)amino]phenyl}acetate)

Bis({4-[bis(2-chloroethyl)amino]benzene}acetate)estra-1,3,5(10)-triene-
3,17-diol(17β); bis({4-[bis(2-chloroethyl)amino]benzene}acetate)oestra-
1,3,5(10)-triene-3,17-diol(17β); bis({*para*[bis(2-chloroethyl)amino]-
phenyl}acetate)estradiol; bis{(*para*[bis(2-chloroethyl)amino]phenyl}-
acetate)estra-1,3,5(10)-triene-3,17β-diol; bis({*para*[bis(2-chloroethyl)-
amino]phenyl}acetate)oestradiol; bis({*para*[bis(2-chloroethyl)amino]-
phenyl}acetate)oestra-1,3,5(10)-triene-3,17β-diol; NSC 112259

1.2   Chemical formula and molecular weight

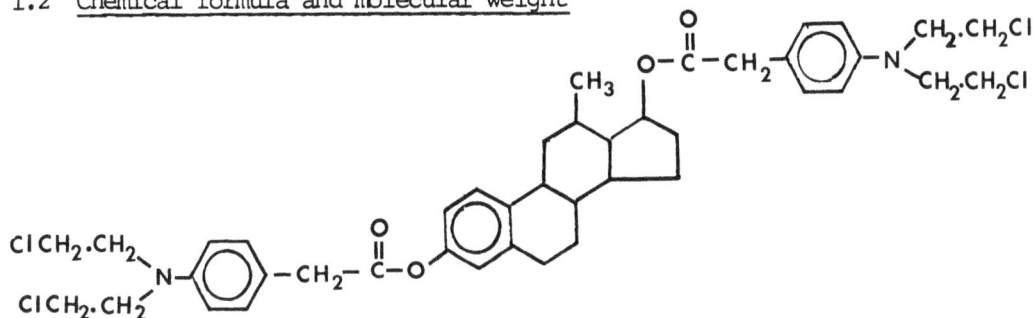

$C_{42}H_{50}Cl_4N_2O_4$

Mol. wt: 788.7

1.3   Chemical and physical properties of the pure substance

(a)   Melting-point: 40-65°C (freeze-dried)

(b)   Spectroscopy data: λ_{max} 261 nm (in ethanol)

(c)   Solubility: Insoluble in water; soluble in dimethyl sulphoxide
and *N*,*N*-dimethylformamide, but addition of water causes precipitation; soluble in benzene, chloroform, ethyl acetate and
2-methoxyethanol

(d) Stability: Solutions in chloroform, benzene, ethyl acetate and
2-methoxyethanol showed no change in 24 hours.

1.4 Technical products and impurities

Oestradiol mustard is not produced commercially.

2. Production, Use, Occurrence and Analysis

For important background information on this section, see preamble,
p. 17.

2.1 Production and use

Oestradiol mustard can be prepared by treating ethyl *para*-aminophenyl-
acetate with ethylene oxide and ethyl alcohol to yield ethyl *para*-[*N,N*-bis-
(2-hydroxyethyl)amino]phenylacetate. This is then chlorinated with phosphorous
oxychloride and hydrolysed to give *para*-[*N,N*-bis(2-chloroethyl)amino]phenyl-
acetic acid. Treatment of this acid with thionyl chloride yields the hydrochloride of *para*-[*N,N*-bis(2-chloroethyl)amino]phenylacetic acid chloride,
which, when treated with oestradiol, yields oestradiol mustard (Wall *et al.*,
1969).

Oestradiol mustard is not manufactured in commercial quantitites in
the US, Europe or Japan. However, both laboratory and clinical studies have
been conducted on its use as an antineoplastic agent. Because both oestrogens
and alkylating agents are believed to produce regressions in mammary tumours
when used separately, trial use of this chemical, which combines both steroid
and mustard moieties, was favoured for advanced breast cancer (Everson *et
al.*, 1973; Vollmer *et al.*, 1973).

2.2 Occurrence

Oestradiol mustard is not known to occur in nature.

2.3 Analysis

Thin-layer chromatography and ultraviolet spectrophotometry may be used
for determination of the pure compound (Vollmer *et al.*, 1973).

218

3. Biological Data Relevant to the Evaluation of Carcinogenic Risk to Man

3.1 Carcinogenicity and related studies in animals

Intraperitoneal administration

Mouse: Male and female A/He mice, 6-8 weeks old, received 8 or 12 i.p. injections of oestradiol mustard in tricaprylin at three dose levels (total doses, 1.6, 1.2 and 0.48 g/kg bw). Two series of controls were maintained: untreated mice killed at the same time as the treated animals, and controls which received the vehicle alone. The experiments were terminated 24 weeks after the first injeciton, and the numbers of treated mice surviving were 19/20, 19/20 and 15/20 at the three dose levels, respectively. Lung tumours developed in 19/19, 19/19 and 11/15 mice, with 5, 3.6 and 2.8 lung tumours per mouse. Of 77 males and 77 females injected with tricaprylin alone and surviving 24 weeks, 28% males and 20% females developed lung tumours, with 0.24 and 0.2 lung tumours per mouse. In the same experiment oestradiol mustard was reported to be about 25 times less potent than uracil mustard on a molar basis (Stoner et al., 1973).

3.2 Other relevant biological data

Daily doses of 20-80 mg/kg bw oestradiol mustard given to dogs for 14 days produced vomiting, lymphopaenia and reversible anaemia at lower doses, and,in addition to these symptoms, convulsions, death and neutropaenia at the highest dose. Female dogs showed signs of oestrus and endometrial hyperplasia; degenerative changes in spermatogenic cells and squamous metaplasia of the prostate were observed in males (Schaeppi et al., 1973).

Oestradiol mustard inhibited the specific binding of ^{3}H-oestradiol-17β to uterine cytosol receptors; the alkylating moiety, phenester[*], was without effect. Sucrose gradient analysis indicated that oestradiol mustard blocked the formation of the specific 8S ^{3}H-oestradiol-17β-receptor complex of cytoplasm(Everson et al., 1974).

---

[*] {para-[bis(2-chloroethyl)amino]phenyl}acetic acid, ethyl ester

3.3 Observations in man

No data were available to the Working Group.

4. Comments on Data Reported and Evaluation[1]

4.1 Animal data

Oestradiol mustard is carcinogenic in mice following its intraperitoneal injection, the only species and route tested, producing a dose-related increase in the incidence of lung tumours.

4.2 Human data

No case reports or epidemiological studies were available to the Working Group.

---

[1] See also the section, "Animal Data in Relation to the Evaluation of Risk to Man" in the introduction to this volume, p. 15.

5. References

Everson, R.B., Hall, T.C. & Wittliff, J.L. (1973) Treatment *in vivo* of R3230AC carcinoma of the rat with estradiol mustard (NSC-112259) or its molecular components. Cancer Chemother. Rep., 57, 353-355

Everson, R.B., Turnell, R.W., Wittliff, J.L. & Hall, T.C. (1974) Estradiol mustard (NSC-112259) and phenester (NSC-116785): possible mediation of action by estrogen binding protein. Cancer Chemother. Rep., 58, 353-358

Schaeppi, U., Heyman, I.A., Fleischman, R.W., Rosenkrantz, H., Ilievski, V., Phelan, R., Cooney, A. & Davis, R.D. (1973) Toxicity in beagle dogs of three alkylating esters with antitumor activity: phenesterin (NSC-104469), estradiol mustard (NSC-112259) and dehydroepiandrosterone mustard (NSC-121210). Cancer Chemother. Rep., Part 3, 4, 85

Stoner, G.D., Shimkin, M.B., Kniazeff, A.J., Weisburger, J.H., Weisburger, E.K. & Gori, G.B. (1973) Test for carcinogenicity of food additives and chemotherapeutic agents by the pulmonary tumor response in strain A mice. Cancer Res., 33, 3069-3085

Vollmer, E.P., Taylor, D.J., Masnyk, I.J., Cooney, D., Levine, B. & Piczak, C. (1973) Estradiol mustard (NSC-112259) - clinical brochure. Cancer Chemother. Rep., Part 3, 4, 121-140

Wall, M.E., Abernethy, G.S., Jr, Carroll, F.I. & Taylor, D.J. (1969) The effects of some steroidal alkylating agents on experimental animal mammary tumor and leukemia systems. J. med. Chem., 12, 810-818

PHENOXYBENZAMINE (HYDROCHLORIDE)

1. Chemical and Physical Data

Phenoxybenzamine

1.1 Synonyms and trade names

Chem. Abstr. Reg. Serial No.: 59-96-1

Chem. Abstr. Name: *N*-(2-Chloroethyl)-*N*-(1-methyl-2-phenoxyethyl)-benzenemethanamine

N-(2-Chloroethyl)-*N*-(1-methyl-2-phenoxyethyl)benzylamine; dibenylin; dibenzylene; *N*-phenoxyisopropyl-*N*-benzyl-β-chloroethylamine

1.2 Chemical formula and molecular weight

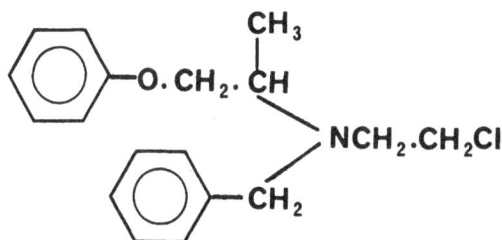

$C_{18}H_{22}ClNO$

Mol. wt: 303.8

1.3 Chemical and physical properties of the pure substance

(a) Description: Crystals from petroleum ether

(b) Melting-point: 38-40°C

(c) Solubility: Soluble in acidified aqueous solutions of propylene glycol; soluble in benzene, heptane and tricaprylin

1.4 Technical products and impurities

Phenoxybenzamine is not manufactured commercially.

Phenoxybenzamine hydrochloride

1.1 Synonyms and trade names

Chem. Abstr. Reg. Serial No.: 63-92-3

Chem. Abstr. Name: N-(2-Chloroethyl)-N-(1-methyl-2-phenoxyethyl)-benzenemethanamine hydrochloride

2-(N-Benzyl-2-chloroethylamino)-1-phenoxypropane hydrochloride;
benzyl(2-chloroethyl)(1-methyl-2-phenoxyethyl)amine hydrochloride;
N-(2-chloroethyl)-N-(1-methyl-2-phenoxyethyl)benzylamine hydrochloride

Bensylyt NEN; Blocadren; Dibenyline; Dibenzyline; Phenoxybenzamin

1.2 Chemical formula and molecular weight

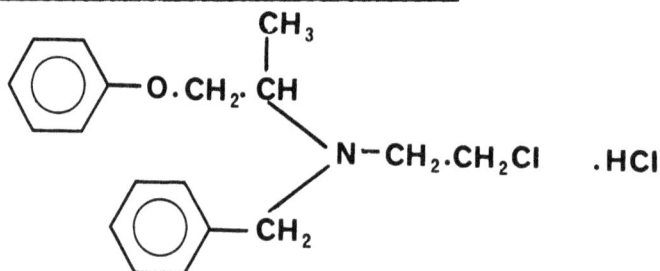

$C_{18}H_{22}ClNO.HCl$ Mol. wt: 340.3

1.3 Chemical and physical properties of the pure substance

(a) Description: A white, odourless, almost tasteless crystalline powder

(b) Melting-point: 137.5-140°C

(c) Spectroscopy data: λ_{max} 272 nm, E_1^1 = 56.3; λ_{max} 279 nm, E_1^1 = 46.1

(d) Solubility: Sparingly soluble in water; soluble in 9 parts ethanol and in 9 parts chloroform; soluble in 50:50 ethanol:propylene glycol

(e) Stability: Solutions in 50:50 ethanol:propylene glycol are stable when stored below 25°C.

1.4 Technical products and impurities

Phenoxybenzamine hydrochloride is available in capsules containing 10 mg active ingredient (Blacow, 1967; Bundesverbrand der pharmazeutischen Industrie, 1969; Pullam, 1968-69; Smith Kline & French Laboratories, 1974).

2. Production, Use, Occurrence and Analysis

For important background information on this section, see preamble, p. 17.

Phenoxybenzamine

2.1 Production and use

Phenoxybenzamine can be prepared by treating 2-phenoxy-1-methyl ethanol with thionyl chloride to yield 2-phenoxy-1-methyl-1-chloroethane. This product is then treated with ethanolamine followed by benzyl chloride to produce the *N*-benzyl derivative. Subsequent treatment with thionyl chloride yields phenoxybenzamine hydrochloride, which can be neutralized to produce phenoxybenzamine (Kerwin & Ullyot, 1954).

2.2 Occurrence

Phenoxybenzamine is not known to occur in nature.

Phenoxybenzamine hydrochloride

2.1 Production and use

Phenoxybenzamine hydrochloride can be prepared by the same method described for phenoxybenzamine. Although it has been produced and marketed by one company in the US since 1953, data on the quantity produced are not reported; it is estimated that sales of phenoxybenzamine hydrochloride in 1973 amounted to approximately 25 kg. It is believed that some of the production was exported to Europe.

This chemical has been used in human medicine as a long-acting adrenergic blocking agent: it is reported to increase peripheral blood flow, raise skin temperature, relieve causalgic pain and lower blood pressure. It has been used to control episodes of hypertension and sweating in phaeochromocytoma and in the treatment of peripheral vascular disorders such as Raynaud's syndrome, acrocyanosis, causalgia, chronic ulceration of the extremities, frostbite sequelae and diabetic gangrene. It has been classified by the US Food and Drug Administration as effective for the treatment of phaeo-chromocytoma and possibly for peripheral vascular disorders. It is adminis-tered orally, in initial doses of 10 mg daily, increasing to 20-60 mg/day, depending on the response of the patient (Medical Economics Company, 1975).

225

2.2 Occurrence

Phenoxybenzamine hydrochloride is not known to occur in nature.

2.3 Analysis

An IR spectrophotometric method for determination of the purity of phenoxybenzamine hydrochloride samples is given in the British Pharmacopoeia (British Pharmacopoeia Commission, 1973). Phenoxybenzamine hydrochloride can be separated by thin-layer chromatography (Masuoka *et al*., 1967).

3. Biological Data Relevant to the Evaluation of Carcinogenic Risk to Man

3.1 Carcinogenicity and related studies in animals

Intraperitoneal administration

Mouse: Three groups of 20 A/He mice of both sexes, 6-8 weeks old, were given 4 i.p. injections of phenoxybenzamine dissolved in tricaprylin for total doses of 200, 100 and 40 mg/kg bw (injection interval not specified). Twenty-four weeks after the first injection the 7, 14 and 20 survivors were killed, and 3, 9 and 9 had lung adenomas and adenocarcinomas, with averages of 0.71, 0.79 and 0.45 tumours per mouse. In controls, 80 mice of each sex received 24 weekly injections of tricaprylin. Of the 77 male and 77 female survivors in each group, lung tumours were found in 28% of males (average, 0.24 tumours/mouse) and 20% of females (average, 0.20 tumours/mouse). [The difference in incidence of lung tumours between treated and control mice was statistically significant at the low ($P<0.05$) and medium ($P<0.01$) dose levels.] In the same experiment, uracil mustard was 46 times more potent than phenoxybenzamine on a molar basis (Stoner *et al*., 1973).

3.2 Other relevant biological data

The oral LD_{50} in rats is 2500 mg/kg bw. In dogs, the lowest lethal i.v. concentration is 10 mg/kg bw. The oral LD_{50} for guinea-pigs is 500 mg/kg bw (Barnes & Eltherington, 1965).

An i.v. injection of ^{14}C-phenoxybenzamine hydrochloride in NMRI mice remained in blood for 40 minutes. Radioactive material was thereafter found in brown fat, liver and kidney; other organs (notably the heart and central nervous system) attained relatively higher activity, which persisted for

4 days. Four hours after i.v. injection of ^{14}C-phenoxybenzamine hydrochloride, the bile from two anaesthetized male Sprague-Dawley rats contained 29.3% and 32.8% of the administered radioactivity (Masuoka *et al.*, 1967).

3.3 Observations in man

No data were available to the Working Group.

4. Comments on Data Reported and Evaluation[1]

4.1 Animal data

Phenoxybenzamine is carcinogenic in mice following its intraperitoneal injection, the only species and route tested, producing an increased incidence of lung tumours.

4.2 Human data

No case reports or epidemiological studies were available to the Working Group.

---

[1] See also the section, "Animal Data in Relation to Evaluation of Risk to Man", in the introduction to this volume, p. 15.

5. References

Barnes, C.D. & Eltherington, L.G. (1965) *Drug Dosages in Laboratory Animals, A Handbook*, Berkeley, University of California Press

Blacow, N.W., ed. (1967) *Martindale: The Extra Pharmacopoeia*, 25th ed., London, The Pharmaceutical Press

British Pharmacopoeia Commission (1973) *British Pharmacopoeia*, London, HMSO, p. 361

Bundesverband der pharmazeutischen Industrie (1969) *Rote Liste*, Frankfurt, p. 940

Kerwin, J.F. & Ullyot, G.E. (1954) *N-(2-Phenoxyisopropyl)ethanolamines. US Patent*, 2,683,719, July 13

Masuoka, D., Appelgren, L.E. & Hansson, E. (1967) Autoradiographic distribution studies of adrenergic blocking agents. I. ^{14}C-Phenoxybenzamine (Bensylyt NFN), an α-receptor-type blocking agent. *Acta pharmacol. (Kbh.)*, 25, 113-122

Medical Economics Company (1975) *Physicians' Desk Reference*, 29th ed., Oradell, NJ, p. 1380

Pullom, E.N., ed. (1968-69) *Mims Annual Compendium*, London, Medical Publications Ltd, p. 304

Smith Kline & French Laboratories (1974) *American Druggist Blue Book: Cumulative Supplement*, October, New York, The Hearst Corporation, p. 401

Stoner, G.D., Shimkin, M.B., Kniazeff, A.J., Weisburger, J.H., Weisburger, E.K. & Gori, G.B. (1973) Test for carcinogenicity of food additives and chemotherapeutic agents by the pulmonary tumor response in strain A mice. *Cancer Res.*, 33, 3069-3085

TRICHLOROTRIETHYLAMINE HYDROCHLORIDE

1. Chemical and Physical Data

1.1 Synonyms and trade names

Chem. Abstr. Reg. Serial No.: 817-09-4

Chem. Abstr. Name: 2-Chloro-N,N-bis(2-chloroethyl)ethanamine hydrochloride

HN3[*]; HN3 hydrochloride; NSC-30211; R-47; SK-100; tri(β-chloroethyl)-amine hydrochloride; 2,2',2"-trichlorotriethylamine hydrochloride; trimustine[*]; trimustine hydrochloride; tris(2-chloroethyl)amine hydrochloride; tris(β-chloroethyl)amine hydrochloride; tris (2-chloroethyl)-amine monohydrochloride; tris(β-chloroethyl)amine monohydrochloride; tris-N-lost; TS-160

Lekamin; Sinalost; Trichlormethine; Trillekamin; Trimitan

1.2 Chemical formula and molecular weight

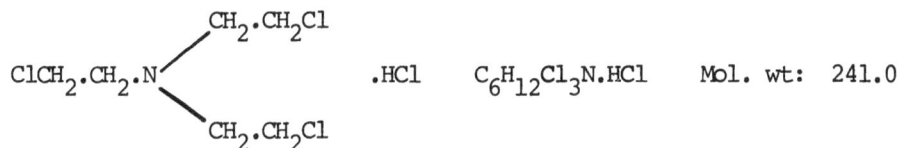

$$\text{ClCH}_2.\text{CH}_2.\text{N} \begin{array}{l} \diagup \text{CH}_2.\text{CH}_2\text{Cl} \\ \diagdown \text{CH}_2.\text{CH}_2\text{Cl} \end{array} \text{.HCl} \quad \text{C}_6\text{H}_{12}\text{Cl}_3\text{N.HCl} \quad \text{Mol. wt: } 241.0$$

1.3 Chemical and physical properties of the pure substance

(a) <u>Description</u>: White powder; the free base is a colourless, oily liquid which becomes yellow or brown on standing.

(b) <u>Melting-point</u>: 131-132.2°C

(c) <u>Solubility</u>: Very soluble in water; soluble in ethanol

(d) <u>Volatility</u>: Volatile at room temperature

(e) <u>Reactivity</u>: Forms picrates

(f) <u>Stability</u>: Aqueous solutions deteriorate rapidly.

---

[*] This name is also used for the free base, trichlorotriethylamine.

1.4 Technical products and impurities

Trichlorotriethylamine hydrochloride is available in Europe in ampoules for i.v. injection containing 5 mg active ingredient mixed with 14 mg citric acid (Bundesverbrand der pharmazeutischen Industrie, 1969).

2. Production, Use, Occurrence and Analysis

For important background information on this section, see preamble, p. 17.

2.1 Production and use

Trichlorotriethylamine hydrochloride can be prepared by treating triethanolamine with thionyl chloride (Ward, 1935).

In the Federal Republic of Germany trichlorotriethylamine hydrochloride is used in human medicine as an antineoplastic agent for the treatment of neoplastic diseases such as lymphogranuloma, lymphosarcoma, giant follicular lymphoma, reticulosarcoma, chronic lymphoid leukaemia, mycosis fungoides, bronchial cancer, Hodgkin's disease, polycythaemia vera and carcinomas of the lung. It is administered intravenously in doses of 1-5 mg at intervals of 2-3 days until a total dose of 20-60 mg has been given (Bundesverbrand der pharmazeutischen Industrie, 1969). Studies of its use as an antineoplastic agent have also been conducted in the US (Bratzel *et al.*, 1963).

Trichlorotriethylamine hydrochloride has also been tested for use in the treatment of arthritis (Vykydal & Klabusay, 1957) and as a fixing agent in textile dyes (Lister *et al.*, 1962, 1964). The corresponding free base, trichlorotriethylamine, is a vesicant but has never been used in military conflict (Witten *et al.*, 1964).

2.2 Occurrence

Trichlorotriethylamine hydrochloride is not known to occur in nature.

2.3 Analysis

A colorimetric method in which 4-(4'-nitrobenzyl)pyridine is used as analytical reagent was applied to assays of various alkylating agents. This chemical may also be determined by thin-layer chromatography (Epstein *et al.*, 1955; Petering & Van Giessen, 1963; Sawicki & Sawicki, 1969).

3. Biological Data Relevant to the Evaluation
of Carcinogenic Risk to Man

3.1 Carcinogenicity and related studies in animals

Subcutaneous, intraperitoneal or intravenous administration

Mouse and rat: A total of 230 Swiss mice and albino rats were injected s.c., i.p. or i.v. with approximately 0.5 mg/kg bw trichlorotriethylamine hydrochloride or methyl-bis(β-chloroethyl)amine hydrochloride. Some animals received a single dose, while others received injections weekly for a period of 5-9 months. Fibrosarcomas, lymphosarcomas and adenocarcinomas (unspecified) developed in 15-20% of the treated animals, whereas no tumours developed in control animals given injections of saline. The tumours usually appeared 4-8 months after administration of the chemicals (Griffin *et al.*, 1950). [No further details were reported.]

3.2 Other relevant biological data

Trichlorotriethylamine hydrochloride is a strong vesicant on skin and causes conjunctivitis and lung damage. The single i.v. LD_{50} for trichlorotriethylamine is 0.7 mg/kg bw for rats and 2.5 mg/kg bw for rabbits; in the case of cutaneous application it was 7 mg/kg bw for mice, 4.9 mg/kg bw for rats, 19 mg/kg bw for rabbits and 1.0 mg/kg bw for dogs (Anslow *et al.*, 1947). Progressive anaemia, lymphocytopaenia and bone-marrow damage were found in mice and rabbits following chronic administration of the hydrochloride. All coloured mice showed greying of hair (Boyland & Horning, 1949; Friederici, 1955).

Trichlorotriethylamine hydrochloride induces point mutations in auxotrophic strains of *Schizosaccharomyces pombe* (Heslot, 1962) and chromosome aberrations in experimental Walker carcinoma cells (Boyland *et al.*, 1948; Koller, 1969).

3.3 Observations in man

No data were available to the Working Group.

4. Comments on Data Reported and Evaluation

4.1 Animal data

Although there is an indication in one study that trichlorotriethyl-amine hydrochloride is carcinogenic in mice and rats, the data are insufficient to allow an evaluation of the carcinogenicity of this chemical.

4.2 Human data

No case reports or epidemiological studies were available to the Working Group.

5. References

Anslow, W.P., Jr, Karnovsky, D.A., Val Jager, B. & Smith, H.W. (1947) The toxicity and pharmacological action of the nitrogen mustards and certain related compounds. J. Pharmacol. exp. Ther., 91, 224-235

Boyland, E. & Horning, E.S. (1949) The induction of tumours with nitrogen mustards. Brit. J. Cancer, 3, 118-123

Boyland, E., Clegg, J.W., Koller, P.C., Rhoden, E. & Warwick, O.H. (1948) The effects of chloroethylamines on tumours, with special reference to bronchogenic carcinoma. Brit. J. Cancer, 2, 17-29

Bratzel, R.P., Ross, R.B., Goodridge, T.H., Huntress, W.T., Flather, M.T. & Johnson, D.E. (1963) Survey of nitrogen mustards. Cancer Chemother. Rep., 26, 1-322

Bundesverband der pharmazeutischen Industrie (1969) Rote Liste, Frankfurt

Epstein, J., Rosenthal, R.W. & Ess, R.J. (1955) Use of γ-(4-nitrobenzyl)-pyridine as analytical reagent for ethyleneimines and alkylating agents. Analyt. Chem., 27, 1435-1439

Friederici, L. (1955) Der Einfluss von Sulfonamiden, Stickstoff-Lost, TEM und Aminopterin auf das Blut und die blutbildenden Organe des Kaninchens. Folia haemat., Lpz., 73, 49-74

Griffin, A.C., Brandt, E.L. & Tatum, E.L. (1950) Nitrogen mustards as cancer-inducing agents. J. Amer. med. Ass., 144, 571

Heslot, H. (1962) Etude quantitative de réversions biochimiques induites chez la levine *Schizosaccharomyces pombe* par des radiations et des substances radiomimétiques. Abh. dtsch. Akad. Wissenschaften (Berl.) klin. Med., 1, 191-228

Koller, P.C. (1969) Mutagenic alkylating agents as growth inhibitors and carcinogens. Mutation Res., 8, 199-206

Lister, G.H., Egli, H. & Ryffel, C. (1962) Dyeing, padding or printing of polyamide fibers. Swiss Patent, 362,051, July 31, Sandoz Ltd

Lister, G.H., Egli, H. & Ryffel, C. (1964) Dyeing and printing of cellulosic textiles. Swiss Patent, 378,280, July 31, Sandoz Ltd

Petering, H.G. & Van Giessen, G.L. (1963) Colorimetric method for determination of uracil mustard and related alkylating agents. J. pharm. Sci., 52, 1159-1162

Sawicki, E. & Sawicki, C.R. (1969) Analysis of alkylating agents: application to air pollution. Ann. N.Y. Acad. Sci., 163, 895-921

Vykydal, M. & Klabusay, L. (1957) Zum Wirkungsmechanismus des *N*-Lost in der experimentellen und klinischen Rheumatologie. <u>Arzneimittel-Forsch.</u>, <u>7</u>, 516-520

Ward, K. (1935) The chlorinated ethylamines - a new type of vesicant. <u>J. Amer. chem. Soc.</u>, <u>57</u>, 914-916

Witten, B., Magaha, E.P. & Williams, W.A. (1964) <u>Chemical warfare.</u> In: Kirk, R.E. & Othmer, D.F., eds, <u>Encyclopedia of Chemical Technology</u>, 2nd ed., Vol. 4, New York, John Wiley and Sons, pp. 871-875

URACIL MUSTARD

1.   Chemical and Physical Data

1.1   Synonyms and trade names

Chem. Abstr. Reg. Serial No.:   66-75-1

Chem. Abstr. Name: 5-[Bis(2-chloroethyl)amino]-2,4(1H,3H)pyrimidine-dione

5-Aminouracil mustard;   5-[bis(2-chloroethyl)amino]uracil;   5-N,N-bis(2-chloroethyl)aminouracil;   CB-4835;   demethyldopan;   desmethyl-dopan;   5-[di(β-chloroethyl)amino]uracil;   2,6-dihydroxy-5-bis(2-chloroethyl)aminopyrimidine;   ENT 50439;   NSC-34462;   SK-19849;   U-8344;   uramustine

1.2   Chemical formula and molecular weight

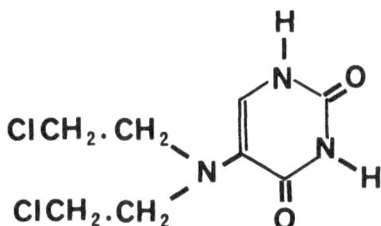

$C_8H_{11}Cl_2N_3O_2$

Mol. wt: 252.1

1.3   Chemical and physical properties of the pure substance

(a)   Description: White, odourless crystals from methanol and water

(b)   Melting-point: About 200°C (decomposition)

(c)   Spectroscopy data: λ_{max} 257 nm (0.01N H_2SO_4 in 95% ethanol); $E_1^1 = 226$

(d)   Solubility: Slightly soluble in methanol and in acetone (2 mg/ml);   very slightly soluble in water;   practically insoluble in benzene and chloroform;   soluble in dimethylacetamide and 5% aqueous solutions thereof

(e) Stability: Unstable in water and acid solutions

1.4 Technical products and impurities

Uracil mustard is available in the US in the form of capsules containing 1 mg active ingredient (Kastrup, 1974).

2. Production, Use, Occurrence and Analysis

For important background information on this section, see preamble,
p. 17.

2.1 Production and use

Uracil mustard can be prepared by treating 5-aminouracil with ethylene
oxide to give 5-bis(2-hydroxyethyl)aminouracil. This product is then
treated with thionyl chloride, yielding uracil mustard (Lyttle & Petering,
1958).

Uracil mustard has been manufactured by one company in the US since
1962; however, only 26 g were manufactured and sold in 1974, and it is
neither imported nor exported by that country.

Uracil mustard has been used in human medicine in the treatment of
various malignant diseases, including chronic lymphocytic leukaemia, follicular lymphomas, Hodgkin's disease, reticulum-cell sarcoma, lymphoblastic
lymphoma, mycosis fungoides, chronic myelogenous leukaemia, polycythaemia
vera and carcinoma of the ovary and lung (Kastrup, 1974). It is administered orally in doses of 1-2 mg daily for three weeks (Goodman & Gilman,
1970).

Uracil mustard has been tested in laboratory animals as an immunosuppressive agent (Buskirk et al., 1965; Karp & Bradley, 1968; Nelson &
Bridges, 1965) and against influenza and vaccinia viruses (Sidwell et al.,
1968) and certain strains of bacteria (Wacker et al., 1966). It has also
been tested as an insect chemosterilant but has never been made commercially
available in the US for this purpose (Fye et al., 1965).

2.2 Occurrence

Uracil mustard is not known to occur in nature.

2.3 Analysis

Uracil mustard may be determined colorimetrically by its reaction with 8-hydroxyquinoline in alkaline solution (Anon., 1964) or by reaction with 4-(4'-nitrobenzyl)pyridine in acid solution for its estimation in blood (Klatt *et al.*, 1960; Petering & Van Giessen, 1963). Both methods can detect about 5 µg/ml.

3. Biological Data Relevant to the Evaluation of Carcinogenic Risk to Man

3.1 Carcinogenicity and related studies in animals

Intraperitoneal administration

Mouse: Three groups of 20 A/He mice of both sexes, 6-8 weeks old, received 7 i.p. injections of uracil mustard in tricaprylin over a 24-week period (total doses, 40, 20 and 8 mg/kg bw). At the end of this period there were 15, 18 and 19 survivors, respectively, and all developed lung adenomas and adenocarcinomas, the averages being 23, 12 and 3.7 tumours per mouse, respectively. In 80 male and 80 female controls which received 24 weekly i.p. injections of tricaprylin, there were 77 male and 77 female survivors at 24 weeks, and 28% males and 20% females developed 0.24 and 0.20 lung tumours per mouse, respectively (Stoner *et al.*, 1973).

Male and female A/J mice, 4-6 weeks old, were given i.p. injections of uracil mustard in tricaprylin or in 1% acacia solution thrice weekly for 4 weeks (total doses ranged from 0.18-12 mg/kg bw). Thirty-nine weeks after the first injection, the survivors were killed and examined for lung adenomas and adenocarcinomas, and the results are shown in the following table (Shimkin *et al.*, 1966):

Total dose (mg/kg bw)	Survivors/ original no. of animals	% Mice with tumours	Mean no. of tumours per mouse
12	28/60	100	15.6
9.6	30/30	100	20.3
3	52/60	100	6.6
0.76	54/60	85	2.0
0.18	55/60	56	0.9
Vehicle (males)	385	39.5	0.5
Vehicle (females)	392	31.4	0.36

Groups of 25 male and 25 female Swiss mice, 6 weeks old, were given i.p. injections of 0.12 or 0.5 mg/kg bw thrice weekly for 6 months, followed by observation for a further 12 months, at which time the animals were killed. Lung tumours occurred in 7/37 males (P=0.1) and in 23/40 females (P<0.001). Liver tumours occurred in 4/37 males (P=0.018) and ovarian tumours and lymphomas occurred in 10/40 and 20/40 females, respectively (P<0.001). The incidences of each tumour type were significantly greater in treated animals than in controls (Weisburger *et al.*, 1975).

Rat: Two groups of 25 male and 25 female Charles River CD rats, 6 weeks old, were given thrice weekly i.p. injections of 0.15 or 0.3 mg/kg bw for 6 months, followed by observation for a further 12 months, at which time the animals were killed. Peritoneal sarcomas occurred in 10/38 males and in 8/39 females (P<0.001); lymphomas occurred in 6/38 males (P<0.001) and in 4/39 females (P=0.004); pancreatic tumours were found in 3/38 males (P=0.005); ovarian tumours and mammary carcinomas were found in 4/39 (P<0.001) and 8/39 (P=0.03) females, respectively. The incidences of each tumour type were significantly greater in treated animals than in controls (Weisburger *et al.*, 1975).

3.2 Other relevant biological data

The oral LD_{50} of uracil mustard in Donryu rats is 3.55 mg/kg bw (Chang, 1964). LD_{50}'s for mice and rats of 2-6 mg/kg bw (orally) and 1-3 mg/kg bw (intramuscularly or intraperitoneally) were reported by Ballerini *et al.* (1965). Chang (1964) found that uracil mustard induced extensive damage in rat bone marrow and testis. In the study of Shimkin *et al.* (1966) quoted above, higher doses of uracil mustard caused hepatic changes consisting of early portal cirrhosis.

$2-^{14}C$-Uracil mustard was administered at a dose of 4 mg to 265 Walker carcinosarcoma-bearing Holzman rats. Incorporation of the ^{14}C-label into macromolecules in subcellular fractions of various tissues was measured for 6 hours after administration and was generally found to be maximal by 1 hour and to be more extensive in RNA than in DNA or protein (Byvoet & Busch, 1962).

Administration of uracil mustard to female rats in doses of 0.3 and 0.6 mg/kg bw on the 12th day of pregnancy produced malformations in the surviving offspring at 21 days: exencephaly, retarded and clubbed appendages and deformed paws and tail were seen (Chaube *et al.*, 1967).

The reaction os 0.2 μmoles/ml uracil mustard with heparinized human blood at $37^{\circ}C$ *in vitro* was measured colorimetrically: about 50% of the original drug was no longer detectable after 30 mins (Klatt *et al.*, 1960).

3.3 <u>Observations in man</u>

No data were available to the Working Group.

4. <u>Comments on Data Reported and Evaluation</u>[1]

4.1 <u>Animal data</u>

Uracil mustard is carcinogenic in mice and rats following its intraperitoneal injection, producing a dose-related increase in the incidence of lung tumours in mice and a variety of tumours in both mice and rats.

4.2 <u>Human data</u>

No case reports or epidemiological studies were available to the Working Group.

---

[1]See also the section, "Animal Data in Relation to the Evaluation of Risk to Man" in the introduction to this volume, p. 15.

5. References

Anon. (1964) Qualitative and quantitative tests for uracil mustard. J. pharm. Sci., 53, 1233-1234

Ballerini, G., Castoldi, G.L., Ricci, N. & Tenze, L. (1965) Experimental and clinical findings on the therapeutic use of a new alkylating agent: uracil mustard. Clin. Terap., 32, 49-61

Buskirk, H.H., Crim, J.A., Petering, H.G., Merritt, K. & Johnson, A.G. (1965) Effect of uracil mustard and several antitumor drugs on the primary antibody response in rats and mice. J. nat. Cancer Inst., 34, 747-758

Byvoet, P. & Busch, H. (1962) Intracellular distribution of 5-bis(2-chloroethyl)aminouracil-2-^{14}C in tissues of tumour bearing rats. Cancer Res., 22, 249-253

Chang, H.S. (1964) Experimental studies on constitution and carcinoma. IX. Pharmacology of uracil mustard as a new chemotherapeutic agent against cancer. Nippon Yakurigaku Zasshi, 60, 413-434

Chaube, S., Kury, G. & Murphy, M.L. (1967) Teratogenic effects of cyclophosphamide (NSC-26271) in the rat. Cancer Chemother. Rep., 51, 363-376

Fye, R.L., Gouck, H.K. & LaBrecque, G.C. (1965) Compounds causing sterility in adult houseflies. J. econ. Entomol., 58, 446-448

Goodman, L.S. & Gilman, A., eds (1970) The Pharmacological Basis of Therapeutics, 4th ed., London, MacMillan, p. 1346

Karp, R.D. & Bradley, S.G. (1968) Effect of immunosuppressive agents on normal phage-neutralizing antibody in the mouse. J. Bact., 96, 1931-1934

Kastrup, E.K., ed. (1974) Facts and Comparisons, St Louis, Missouri, Facts & Comparisons Inc.

Klatt, O., Griffin, A.C. & Stehlin, J.S., Jr (1960) Method for determination of phenylalanine mustard and related alkylating agents in blood. Proc. Soc. exp. Biol. (N.Y.), 104, 629-631

Lyttle, D.A. & Petering, H.G. (1958) 5-Bis(2-chloroethyl)aminouracil, a new antitumor agent. J. Amer. chem. Soc., 80, 6459-6460

Nelson, S.D. & Bridges, J.M. (1965) Effect of uracil mustard on the homograft response in rabbits. Transplantation, 3, 580-581

Petering, H.G. & Van Giessen, G.J. (1963) Colorimetric method for determination of uracil mustard and related alkylating agents. J. pharm. Sci., 52, 1159-1162

240

Shimkin, M.B., Weisburger, J.H., Weisburger, E.K., Gubareff, N. & Suntzeff, V. (1966) Bioassay of 29 alkylating chemicals by the pulmonary tumor response in strain A mice. J. nat. Cancer Inst., 36, 915-935

Sidwell, R.W., Dixon, G.J., Sellers, S.M. & Schabel, F.M., Jr (1968) In vivo antiviral properties of biologically active compounds. II. Studies with influenza and vaccinia viruses. Appl. Microbiol., 16, 370-392

Stoner, G.D., Shimkin, M.B., Kniazeff, A.J., Weisburger, J.H., Weisburger, E.K. & Gori, G.B. (1973) Test for carcinogenicity of food additives and chemotherapeutic agents by the pulmonary tumor response in strain A mice. Cancer Res., 33, 3069-3085

Wacker, A., Kirschfeld, S. & Traeger, L. (1966) The action mechanism of cytostatic thymine analogs in bacteria. Naturwissenschaften, 53, 257-258

Weisburger, J.H., Griswold, D.P., Jr, Prejean, J.D., Casey, A.E., Wood, H.B., Jr & Weisburger, E.K. (1975) The carcinogenic properties of some of the principal drugs used in cancer chemotherapy. Recent Results Cancer Res. (in press)

SELENIUM

SELENIUM AND SELENIUM COMPOUNDS

A WHO Environmental Health Criteria document is in preparation, and therefore the chemical and physical data and information on production, use, occurrence and analysis are covered only briefly. As to the biological data, only those which are strictly relevant to the assessment of carcinogenic risk are mentioned.

1. Chemical and Physical Data

1.1 Synonyms and trade names

Chem. Abstr. Reg. Serial No.:   778-24-92

C.I. No.:   77805

1.2 Chemical identity and atomic weight

Selenium is an element of Group VIA of the periodic table, lying between sulphur and tellurium. Its atomic number is 34 and its atomic weight, 78.96. Selenium has six stable isotopes with mass numbers 74, 76, 77, 78, 80 and 82.

1.3 Chemical and physical properties of the pure substance

(a) Description: Three allotropic modifications exist: (1) monoclinic (red) selenium, m.p. 144°C; (2) grey selenium, m.p. 217°C; and (3) amorphous selenium, which has three forms - vitreous, red amorphous and colloidal selenium.

(b) Solubility: Soluble in carbon disulphide, benzene and quinoline. Selenium oxide is very soluble in water, methanol, ethanol and acetone. Sodium selenite and sodium selenate are also readily soluble in water.

(c) Stability: Oxidized to selenious acid by nitric acid. Amorphous selenium reacts with water to give selenious acid. Selenium oxide, selenites and selenates are easily reduced to selenium. Sodium selenide decomposes in water.

(d) Reactivity: The most important valencies of selenium are Se^{II}, Se^{IV} and Se^{VI}.

Selenium oxychloride, $SeOCl_2$, a yellowish corrosive liquid, attacks most metals and is a solvent for sulphur, selenium, tellurium, rubber, bakelite, gums, resins, celluloid, gelatin, glue, asphalt and other materials. Selenium reacts with metals to gain electrons and to form ionic selenide compounds; covalent compounds are formed with other elements.

1.4 Technical products and impurities

Selenium is available in commercial, high-purity and ultra-high-purity grades. The commercial grade contains a minimum of 99% selenium and may contain maximums of 0.2% tellurium, 0.1% iron, 0.005% lead and 0.005% copper as impurities. It is sold as 200-mesh powder, in lump size and in a size of intermediate coarseness. The high-purity grade, sold in shotted and powder forms, is reported to contain a minimum of 99.99% selenium. Impurities which may be present at concentrations no greater than 1-2 mg/kg each are mercury, tellurium, iron, arsenic and other non-ferrous metals undesirable in electronic and electrostatic applications. Higher concentrations of "inert" contaminants such as sodium, magnesium, calcium, aluminium and silicon can be tolerated. The ultra-high-purity grade, prepared only on a laboratory scale, is reported to contain 0.0001-0.001% impurities. Ferroselenium, containing 57.5% selenium, is also available commercially (Elkin & Margrave, 1968).

2. Production, Use, Occurrence and Analysis

A review on selenium has been published (Elkin & Margrave, 1968).

2.1 Production and use

Selenium was first isolated from pyrite by Berzelius (Berzelius, 1817) as a red sediment in sulphuric acid. Now nearly all selenium is obtained as a by-product of the electrolytic refining of copper, in which copper-refinery slimes are treated with sulphuric acid to dissolve the copper as copper sulphate. In one method used commercially in the United States, de-copperized slimes are smelted in a rotary kiln with sodium bisulphate, and selenium dioxide is volatized and collected in a scrubber-Cottrell system. A small amount of selenium is recovered in the manufacture of sulphuric acid.

246

Purified selenium may be obtained by dissolving the dioxide in water and precipitating selenium with sulphur dioxide (Elkin & Margrave, 1968).

World production of selenium in 1973 was estimated to have been 1.1 million kg (Baltrusaitis, 1974; US Bureau of Mines, 1974); 80% of this was produced in Canada, Japan and the US.

Commercially produced compounds include selenium dioxide, sodium selenite, sodium selenate, selenic acid, selenium oxychloride, cadmium sulphoselenide and selenium diethyldithiocarbamate (Elkin & Margrave, 1968).

Selenium is used in the manufacture of glass to impart red and bronze colours or tints, and to neutralize undesirable green colours produced by iron impurities. The glass container industry consumes 0.11-0.14 million kg of selenium annually (Baltrusaitis, 1974; Elkin & Margrave, 1968).

In the paint, plastics and ceramics industries, cadmium sulphoselenide pigments are used to produce colours ranging from yellow to maroon (Elkin & Margrave, 1968).

Because of its semi-conducting properties, selenium has been used in the manufacture of rectifiers for electronics applications. In recent years, silicon has replaced selenium in high-voltage industrial rectifiers, but selenium rectifiers are still in demand for home-entertainment equipment (Baltrusaitis, 1974). It is also used in photoelectric cells for instruments such as photometers, colorimeters, "electric eyes" and photographic exposure meters (Elkin & Margrave, 1968); and selenium-coated photoreceptors are used more and more frequently in dry photocopiers (Baltrusaitis, 1974).

Selenium is used as an additive to improve the machinability and to reduce the porosity of steels (Baltrusaitis, 1974). It is also used as an additive in both natural and synthetic rubbers to increase the rate of vulcanization and to improve the ageing and mechanical properties of sulphurless and low-sulphur stocks (Elkin & Margrave, 1968).

Selenium sulphide is the active ingredient in several pharmaceutical and cosmetic products, including a prescription drug for the treatment of dandruff and a non-prescription dandruff shampoo, which are used for the treatment of superficial skin mycosis (Baltrusaitis, 1974; Elkin &

247

Margrave, 1968). Approximately 200 kg of this compound are believed to be consumed annually in these products.

Selenium and its compounds are also used as catalysts, e.g., in laboratory determinations of nitrogenous materials and as oxidizing agents in the synthesis of certain organic chemicals such as cortisone and niacin (Elkin & Margrave, 1968), and as reducing agents. Selenium diethyldithiocarbamate has also been reported to have been used as a fungicide (Innes *et al.*, 1969).

In 1974 the US Food and Drug Administration approved the use of sodium selenite or selenate in the feeds of swine, turkeys and growing chickens up to 16 weeks of age; the permissible levels are 0.1 mg/kg in swine and chicken feeds and 0.2 mg/kg in turkey feeds (Anon., 1974). The purpose of these additives in feed is to prevent selenium deficiencies, which can result in decreased growth rates, disease and death (Anon., 1973). The nutritional value of the selenium found in trace amounts in the human diet has also been studied (Higgs *et al.*, 1972).

In veterinary medicine, selenium salts have been used in conjunction with vitamin E to prevent muscular dystrophy. Sodium selenate has been administered to prevent exudative diathesis in chicks, white muscle disease in sheep and infertility in ewes. It is reported to prevent pneumonia in premature lambs and calves and to control hepatitis in swine (Elkin & Margrave, 1968).

2.2 Occurrence

Selenium is widely distributed throughout the environment, occurring in air, water, soil, vegetation and food.

It occurs in metal sulphide deposits that are mined primarily for copper, zinc, nickel and silver. The burning of coal represents the principal source of environmental contamination with selenium compounds: estimates of the amount of selenium released annually to the atmosphere in the US in this way are of up to 4 million kg.

Selenium is present in the major oceans and in inland waters; as a result, it occurs in drinking-water.

Its presence in soil in varying concentrations contributes to its occurrence in many plants some of which absorb and accumulate large amounts of this element. Selenium can occur in paper and paper products and is subsequently released to air upon their incineration.

Due to its widespread occurrence, it is found in animals and foods. Major dietary sources of selenium are meats, fish, dairy products, cereal products and bread.

2.3 Analysis

A wide variety of techniques have been successfully employed for the analysis of selenium in atmospheric samples and in coal, fuel, oil, petrol, biological materials, water sediments and soil samples. These include neutron activation analysis (limit of detection, 0.01 µg/l of air) (Hashimoto & Winchester, 1967); gas absorption followed by spectrophotometry (Kawamura & Matsumoto, 1965) (limit of detection, 150 ng/g coal) (Weaver, 1973); flameless atomic absorption (limit of detection, less than 10 µg/l water) (Baird et $al.$, 1972); atomic absorption spectrometry (limit of detection, 1.3 mg/kg) (Kirkbright & Ronson, 1971); spark source mass spectrometry (von Lehmden et $al.$, 1974); polarography (limit of detection, 0.2 µg/l-2 g biological sample) (Christian et $al.$, 1965); emission spectrometry (limit of detection, 0.02 µg/g fuel oil) (von Lehmden et $al.$, 1974); X-ray fluorescence (Brar et $al.$, 1970); gas chromatography (Burgett, 1974); and high-pressure liquid chromatography (limit of detection, 0.5 mg/l) (Wheeler & Lott, 1974). A critical evaluation of analytical methods for the determination of selenium was made by Shendrikar (1974).

The best methods are neutron activation analysis or fluorometry. Sub-microgram amounts of selenium in a large number of biological samples have been determined fluorometrically (Watkinson, 1966), and this method is being adopted for use as a standard method by the American Association of Agricultural Chemists. A modification of the official method for estimating selenium in plants was reported by Olson et $al.$ (1975).

Selenium can be determined spectrophotometrically or fluorometrically as the selenodiazole complex, following wet oxidation (Hoste & Gills, 1955).

3. Biological Data Relevant to the Evaluation of Carcinogenic Risk to Man

The problem of selenium and cancer has been reviewed (Anon., 1970; Scott, 1973; Shapiro, 1972).

3.1 Carcinogenicity and related studies in animals

Oral administration

Mouse: Administration of either sodium selenite or sodium selenate in drinking-water (to give concentrations of 3 mg/l selenium) to two groups of about 100 Swiss mice of both sexes had little effect on growth rate. Of 88 treated mice examined, 13 (15%) had tumours, compared with 23 (19%) among 119 controls. In the selenium-fed mice, there were 8 "lymphoma-leukaemias", 4 lung adenocarcinomas and 1 osteosarcoma. In the controls there were 2 "lymphoma-leukaemias", 7 lung carcinomas, 1 carcinoma of unknown origin and 13 benign tumours of breast, ovary and other tissues. All of the tumours occurring in the selenium group were malignant, while only 10/23 of the tumours occurring in control animals were malignant (Schroeder & Mitchener, 1972). [The higher incidence of malignancy in the selenium groups was not significant.]

Two groups of 18 male and 18 female mice of the $(C57Bl/6xC3H/Anf)F_1$ or $(C57Bl/6xAKR)F_1$ strain were given daily doses of 10 mg/kg bw ethyl selenac (selenium diethyldithiocarbamate) by gavage, starting when the animals were 7 days of age, until they were 28 days of age. Subsequently, ethyl selenac was given at a level of 26 mg/kg of diet, and feeding was continued for up to 82 weeks. Tumours were induced in 16/18 male (12 hepatomas, 3 lymphomas and 1 sebaceous gland adenoma) and in 6/17 female (3 hepatomas, 2 lymphomas and 1 mammary carcinoma) mice of the $(C57Bl/6xC3H/Anf)F_1$ strain and in 5/17 male (3 hepatomas, 1 lymphoma and 3 pulmonary tumours) and 4/17 female (3 lymphomas and 1 pulmonary tumour) mice of the $(C57Bl/6xAKR)F_1$ strain. The increased incidence of hepatomas over that found in controls was significant (P=0.01) in $(C57Bl/6xC3H/Anf)F_1$ males (Innes et al., 1969; National Technical Information Service, 1968).

[In the same experiment (National Technical Information Service, 1968), a similar fungicide not containing selenium, i.e., potassium bis(2-hydroxy-ethyl)dithiocarbamate, given at a daily dose of 464 mg/kg bw and then at 112 mg/kg of diet, induced a similar incidence of tumours; thus, the tumours may have been caused by the thiocarbamate residue rather than by selenium. On the other hand, feeding of 46.4 mg/kg bw tellurium diethyl-dithiocarbamate followed by 149 mg/kg of diet produced fewer tumours, and feeding of 100 mg/kg bw of the zinc salt followed by 260 mg/kg of diet did not increase the incidence of tumours.]

Rat: Six groups each of 18 female Osborne-Mendel rats were fed seleniferous corn or wheat to give concentrations of 5, 7 or 10 mg selenium per kg of diet, and one group was fed a mixed solution of ammonium potassium sulphide and ammonium potassium selenide to give 10 mg selenium per kg of diet. Of rats surviving between 18-24 months 11/53 developed liver-cell tumours reported as ranging from adenomas to low-grade carcinomas. Only 4 rats receiving 10 mg/kg selenium lived for 2 years. Advanced adenomatoid hyperplasia was seen in 4 rats. Cirrhosis of the liver was present in 43/53 animals, and liver tumours occurred only in animals with cirrhosis. No liver tumours were seen in 73 rats which survived less than 18 months, although cirrhosis was frequent after 3 months. The spontaneous incidence of hepatic tumours in control rats and in rats used in other experiments was reported to be less than 1%; these animals received a diet containing 12% protein and consisting of 49% corn, 44% wheat and 3% yeast (Nelson *et al*., 1943).

Groups of about 100 male and female weanling Long-Evans rats were given 2 mg/l selenium as sodium selenite or sodium selenate in drinking-water (equivalent to about 4.5 mg/kg of diet) until they were 1 year of age when the dose was raised to 3 mg/l. A group of 105 controls received no selenium in drinking-water. After 58 days male rats receiving 2 mg/l sodium selenite were transferred to sodium selenate, since 50% of the animals had died; surviving animals in this group were killed after 596 days and no tumours were observed. Thirty tumours were reported in the 48 selenate-treated rats examined histologically (62.5%); 20 of these tumours were malignant (41.7%). In 32 female selenite-treated rats killed between 662-691 days, 4 malignant tumours were found (12.5%).

Of the 65 control rats examined, 20 had tumours (30.8%) 11 of which were malignant (16.9%). Malignant tumours occurring in both treated and control animals were mainly mammary carcinomas, sarcomas at various sites and "lymphoma-leukaemias" (Schroeder & Mitchener, 1971a). [Although there is a statistical difference in the incidence of all tumours and that of malignant tumours between control and selenate-treated groups, an evaluation of these results was not possible because not all autopsied animals were examined histologicallly and because treated animals lived longer than controls (the average lifespan of control males and females was 813 and 814 days and that of treated animals 847 and 929 days, respectively).]

Wistar rats fed selenium at concentrations of 4, 6, 8 or 16 mg/kg of diet (added as selenite or selenate) died with toxic hepatitis within 100 days. Of 275 rats fed 0.5 or 2 mg/kg of diet, 2 developed lymphomas, 2, mammary adenocarcinomas and 4, other neoplasms within 448-647 days. Of 230 controls, 1 developed a lymphoma, 6, mammary adenocarcinomas and 3, other tumours within 356-613 days. No liver tumours were observed (Harr *et al.*, 1967).

3.2 Other relevant biological data

In animals selenium is both an essential trace element and a naturally occurring toxicant, manifesting high biological activity: it is necessary to sustain life at dietary levels of μg/kg; it is toxic at dietary levels comparable to the nutritional requirements for some other trace elements (Underwood, 1971).

The toxicity of different forms of selenium has been determined by Franke & Moxon (1936, 1937). Sodium selenate is less toxic than the selenite (Schroeder & Mitchener, 1971a). For sodium selenite, the oral LD_{50} in mice is 7-10.5 mg/kg bw (Pletnikova, 1970); the i.v. LD_{50} in rats is 3 mg/kg bw (Stecher, 1968). Acute toxic effects of selenium have been summarized by Underwood (1971); they include degeneration of liver, kidneys and myocardia, haemorrhagia in the digestive tract and brain damage.

Gastrointestinal absorption of selenium, its retention, distribution within the body and excretion vary with species and the amount and chemical form of selenium ingested. Under physiological conditions, animals rapidly excrete most of an administered dose of selenium. Following its absorption, it is transported by albumin to more stable binding sites in blood and tissues. The kidney (particularly the cortex) retains the highest concentration of selenium, followed by the glandular tissues, especially pancreas, pituitary and liver (Underwood, 1971).

Several selenium-deficiency disturbances sometimes associated with vitamin E deficiency are naturally-occurring diseases and have been induced experimentally in laboratory animals. Selenium is generally considered to act in a way which parallels the antioxidant properties of vitamin E. The active form of selenium may be selenide, located in non-haem iron-containing proteins; the function of vitamin E may be to protect the selenide from oxidation (Caygill *et al.*, 1971; Diplock, 1970).

Postulated mechanisms for the biochemical activity of selenium are: (1) as an antioxidant; (2) as a radical scavenger; (3) as a redox substance; (4) in enzyme systems; (5) in the stabilization of membranes (e.g., lysosome membranes); and (6) in the mimicking of processes involving sulphur.

Selenium crosses the placenta in mice, rats, dogs and sheep (Underwood, 1971); it produces runting in mice and premature death in young mice and rats (Schroeder & Mitchener, 1971b).

When single doses of 125 mg 7,12-dimethylbenzanthracene (DMBA) in acetone were applied to the skin of Swiss albino ICR mice, followed 3 weeks later by painting with croton oil containing 0.5 mg/l sodium selenide on 5 days a week for 16 weeks, the incidence of skin tumours was much lower in mice receiving croton oil plus selenium, compared with that in mice receiving croton oil alone (Shamberger & Rudolph, 1966). Similar results were obtained following skin application of DMBA with croton oil, croton resin, 12-tetradecanoyl-phorbol-13-acetate or phenol (Riley, 1968; Shamberger, 1970).

In groups of female Swiss albino ICR mice fed selenium-deficient Torula yeast diets containing 0, 0.1 or 1 mg/kg sodium selenite followed by a single skin painting with 0.125 mg DMBA in acetone and application of croton oil to the skin daily for 20 weeks, the incidence of skin tumours in the group fed 1 mg/kg sodium selenite was lower. Similar results

253

were obtained in groups of mice fed these diets before the application of
0.25 ml of a 0.03% solution of benzo(a)pyrene in acetone to the shaved
skin daily for 27 weeks (Shamberger, 1970).

The incidence of liver tumours in rats fed 3'-methyl-4-dimethylamino-
azobenzene (3'-Me-DAB) for 20 weeks was 12/23, compared with 6/22 in
animals fed 5 mg sodium selenite per kg of diet plus 3'-Me-DAB (Clayton &
Baumann, 1949).

Administration of 2 mg/l selenium oxide in drinking-water to virgin
female C3H/St mice for 15 months lowered the incidence of spontaneous
mammary tumours to 10% from an observed incidence of 82% in untreated
controls (Schrauzer & Ishmael, 1974).

Four groups of 20 female OSU-Brown rats were fed 150 mg N-2-fluorenyl-
acetamide per kg of diet plus 2.5, 0.5, 0.1 or 0 mg selenium per kg of
diet. Incidences of mammary adenocarcinomas and/or hepatic carcinomas
at 200 days were 0/20, 2/20, 12/20 and 12/20, respectively (Harr et $al.$,
1972).

Selenium significantly reduced the chromosome breakage induced by
DMBA in human leucocytes cultured in $vitro$ (Shamberger et $al.$, 1973a).

Pharmacological and toxicological effects of selenium in man have been
reviewed by various authors (Glover, 1970; Rosenfeld & Beath, 1964;
Schroeder et $al.$, 1970; Smith & Westfall, 1937). Acute toxic effects
following exposure to selenium dioxide involve the lungs, stomach and skin;
damage to the digestive tract, nails and teeth have also been described
following its oral administration (Schroeder et $al.$, 1970). An inverse
relationship between selenium occurrence at environmental levels
and the American neonatal death rate has been reported (Shamberger, 1971).
Selenium occurs in blood at a level of about 200 µg/l (Shamberger et $al.$,
1973b).

3.3 Observations in man

Shamberger & Frost (1969) and Shamberger & Willis (1971) have claimed
a negative correlation between cancer mortality and selenium levels in
human blood and in animal foodstuffs. Shamberger & Willis (1971) examined

the total cancer mortality rates (some, but not all, age-adjusted) in the 19 US cities for which Allaway *et al.* (1968) had reported blood selenium levels, and a negative correlation was found. This negative correlation depended for its statistical significance on the presence of data for two cities, Rapid City and Cheyenne, where the blood selenium levels were highest; without these data no correlation was evident. These workers also examined mortality data for the years 1959-61 for cancer at many sites in both sexes in 17 large and 20 small cities in areas from which high selenium levels in animal forage foodstuffs had been reported, and similarly in 17 large and 20 small cities in 'low selenium' areas. No consistent differences were evident in either sex from national rates for US metropolitan cities in either area, although there was a tendency for the rates for certain cancer sites to be lower in cities in the 'high selenium' areas than in the 'low' areas. More recently, age-adjusted mortality rates for certain cancers have been reported to be lower in two Canadian provinces with low selenium levels in animal forage foodstuffs than in six 'high selenium' provinces (Shamberger *et al.*, 1974). In this connection, it is relevant that the population of the two 'low' provinces is more rural than the larger population of the six 'high' provinces.

Shamberger *et al.* (1973b) found that mean selenium blood levels were lower in patients with certain cancers such as those of stomach and colon than in a control group, although this difference was not observed in breast or rectum cancer patients. The only known occupational study of workers exposed to selenium is that reported by Glover (1970) of 300 workers followed for up to 26 years. No differences were detected in the observed as compared to the expected numbers of deaths either from all causes or from cancer.

4. Comments on Data Reported and Evaluation

4.1 Animal data

Selenium compounds were tested in mice and rats by the oral route. Although in one experiment in rats selenium produced an increase in the incidence of liver tumours, the available data are insufficient to allow an evaluation of the carcinogenicity of selenium compounds.

4.2 Human data

The available data provide no suggestion that selenium is carcinogenic in man, and the evidence for a negative correlation between regional cancer death rates and selenium is not convincing.

5. References

Allaway, W.H., Kubota, J., Losee, F. & Roth, M. (1968) Selenium, molybdenum, and vanadium in human blood. Arch. environm. Hlth, 16, 342-348

Anon. (1970) Selenium and cancer. Nutr. Rev., 28, 75-80

Anon. (1973) Selenium feed usage to be allowed by FDA. Chemical Marketing
Reporter, May 7, pp. 7, 23

Anon. (1974) Selenium approved. Agriscience, January 23, p. 1

Baird, R.B., Pourian, S. & Gabrielian, S.M. (1972) Determination of trace
amounts of selenium in wastewaters by carbon rod atomization.
Analyt. Chem., 44, 1887-1889

Baltrusaitis, V.A. (1974) Selenium - production falls short of growing
demand. Engineering and Mining Journal, March, pp. 134-135

Berzelius, J.J. (1817) Sur deux metaux nouveaux (litium et selenium).
Schweigger J., 21, 1818-1823

Brar, S.S., Nelson, D.M., Kline, J.R., Gustafson, P.F., Kanabrocki, E.L.,
Moore, C.E. & Hattori, D.M. (1970) Instrumental analysis for trace
elements present in Chicago area surface air. J. geophys. Res., 75,
2939-2945

Burgett, C.A. (1974) The gas chromatography of selenium as the trimethyl
silyl derivative. Analyt. Letters, 7, 799-806

Caygill, C.P.J., Lucy, J.A. & Diplock, A.T. (1971) The effect of vitamin E
on the intracellular distribution of the different oxidation states
of selenium in rat liver. Biochem. J., 125, 407

Christian, G.D., Knoblock, E.C. & Purdy, W.C. (1965) Polarographic
determination of selenium in biological materials. J. Ass. off.
agric. Chem., 48, 877-884

Clayton, C.C. & Baumann, C.A. (1949) Diet and azo dye tumors: effect of
diet during a period when the dye is not fed. Cancer Res., 9, 575-582

Diplock, A.T. (1970) Recent studies on the interactions between vitamin E
and selenium. In: Mills, C.F., ed., Trace Element Metabolism in
Animals, Edinburgh, E. & S. Livingstone, pp. 190-204

Elkin, E.M. & Margrave, J.L. (1968) Selenium. In: Kirk, R.E. & Othmer,
D.F., eds, Encyclopedia of Chemical Technology, 2nd ed., Vol. 17,
New York, John Wiley & Sons, pp. 809-833

Franke, K.W. & Moxon, A.L. (1936) A comparison of the minimum fatal doses of selenium, tellurium, arsenic and vanadium. J. Pharmacol. exp. Ther., 58, 454-459

Franke, K.W. & Moxon, A.L. (1937) The toxicity of orally ingested arsenic, selenium, tellurium, vanadium and molybdenum. J. Pharmacol. exp. Ther., 61, 89-102

Glover, J.R. (1970) Selenium and its industrial toxicology. Industr. Med., 39, 50-54

Harr, J.R., Bone, J.F., Tinsley, I.J., Weswig, P.H. & Yamamoto, R.S. (1967) Selenium toxicity in rats. II. Histopathology. In: Muth, O.H., ed., Selenium in Bio-Medicine, Westport, Connecticut, Avi Publishing Company, pp. 153-178

Harr, J.R., Exon, J.H., Whanger, P.D. & Weswig, P.H. (1972) Effect of dietary selenium on N-2-fluorenyl-acetamide (FAA)-induced cancer in vitamin E supplemented, selenium depleted rats. Clin. Toxicol., 5, 187-194

Hashimoto, Y. & Winchester, J.W. (1967) Selenium in the atmosphere. Environm. Sci. Technol., 1, 338-340

Higgs, D.J., Morris, V.C. & Levander, O.A. (1972) Effect of cooking on selenium content of foods. J. agric. Fd Chem., 20, 678-679

Hoste, J. & Gills, J. (1955) Spectrophotometric determination of traces of selenium with diaminobenzidine. Analyt. chim. acta, 12, 158-161

Innes, J.R.M., Ulland, B.M., Valerio, M.G., Petrucelli, L., Fishbein, L., Hart, E.R., Pallotta, A.J., Bates, R.R., Falk, H.L., Gart, J.J., Klein, M., Mitchell, I. & Peters, J. (1969) Bioassay of pesticides and industrial chemicals for tumorigenicity in mice: A preliminary note. J. nat. Cancer Inst., 42, 1101-1114

Kawamura, M. & Matsumoto, K. (1965) Determination of small amounts of hydrogen selenide in the air. Bunseki Kagaku, 14, 789-795

Kirkbright, G.F. & Ronson, L. (1971) Use of the nitrous oxide-acetylene flame for determination of arsenic and selenium by atomic absorption spectrometry. Analyt. Chem., 43, 1238-1241

von Lehmden, D.J., Jungers, R.H. & Lee, R.E., Jr (1974) Determination of trace elements in coal, fly ash, fuel oil and gasoline: a preliminary comparison of selected analytical techniques. Analyt. Chem., 43, 239-245

National Technical Information Service (1968) Evaluation of Carcinogenic, Teratogenic and Mutagenic Activities of Selected Pesticides and Industrial Chemicals, Vol. 1, Carcinogenic Study, Washington DC, US Department of Commerce

Nelson, A.A., Fitzhugh, O.G. & Calvery, H.O. (1943) Liver tumors following cirrhosis caused by selenium in rats. Cancer Res., 3, 230-236

Olson, O.E., Palmer, I.S. & Cary, E.E. (1975) Modification of the official fluorometric method for selenium in plants. J. Ass. off. analyt. Chem., 58, 117-121

Pletnikova, I.P. (1970) Biological action and the non-injuriousness level of selenium when it enters the organism together with drinking water. Gig. i Sanit., 35, 14-19

Riley, J.F. (1968) Mast cells, co-carcinogenesis and anti-carcinogenesis in the skin of mice. Experientia, 15, 1237-1238

Rosenfeld, I. & Beath, O.A. (1964) Selenium, New York, Academic Press, p. 279

Schrauzer, G.N. & Ishmael, D. (1974) Effects of selenium and of arsenic on the genesis of spontaneous mammary tumors in inbred C3H mice. Ann. clin. lab. Sci., 4, 441-447

Schroeder, H.A. & Mitchener, M. (1971a) Selenium and tellurium in rats: effects on growth, survival and tumors. J. Nutr., 101, 1531-1540

Schroeder, H.A. & Mitchener, M. (1971b) Toxic effects of trace elements on the reproduction of mice and rats. Arch. environm. Hlth, 23, 102-106

Schroeder, H.A. & Mitchener, M. (1972) Selenium and tellurium in mice: effects on growth, survival and tumors. Arch. environm. Hlth, 24, 66-71

Schroeder, H.A., Frost, D.V. & Belassa, J.J. (1970) Essential trace metals in man: selenium. J. chron. Dis., 23, 227-243

Scott, M.L. (1973) The selenium dilemma. J. Nutr., 103, 803-810

Shamberger, R.J. (1970) Relationship of selenium to cancer. I. Inhibitory effect of selenium on carcinogenesis. J. nat. Cancer Inst., 44, 931-936

Shamberger, R.J. (1971) Is selenium a teratogen? Lancet, ii, 1316

Shamberger, R.J. & Frost, D.V. (1969) Possible protective effect of selenium against human cancer. Canad. med. Ass. J., 100, 682

Shamberger, R.J. & Rudolph, G. (1966) Protection against cocarcinogenesis by antioxidants. Experientia, 22, 116

Shamberger, R.J. & Willis, C.E. (1971) Selenium distribution and human cancer mortality. CRC crit. Rev. clin. lab. Sci., 2, 211-221

Shamberger, R.J., Banghman, F.F., Kalchert, S.L., Willis, C.E. & Hoffman, G.C. (1973a) Carcinogen-induced chromosomal breakage decreased by antioxidants. Proc. nat. Acad. Sci. (Wash.), 70, 1461-1463

Shamberger, R.J., Rukovena, E., Longfield, A.K., Tytko, S.A., Deodhar, S. & Willis, C.E. (1973b) Antioxidants and cancer. I. Selenium in the blood of normal and cancer patients. J. nat. Cancer Inst., 50, 863-870

Shamberger, R.J., Tytko, S. & Willis, C. (1974) Antioxidants and cancer. II. Selenium distribution and human cancer mortality in the United States, Canada and New Zealand. In: Hemphill, D.D., ed., Trace Substances in Environmental Health, Columbia, Missouri, University of Missouri, pp. 31-34

Shapiro, J.R. (1972) Selenium and carcinogenesis: a review. Ann. N.Y. Acad. Sci., 192, 215-219

Shendrikar, A.D. (1974) Critical evaluation of analytical methods for the determination of selenium in air, water and biological materials. Sci. total Environm., 3, 155-169

Smith, M.I. & Westfall, B.B. (1937) Further field studies on the selenium problem in relation to public health. US publ. Hlth Rep., 52, 1375-1384

Stecher, P.G., ed. (1968) The Merck Index, 8th ed., Rahway, N.J., Merck & Co., p. 965

Underwood, E.J. (1971) Trace Elements in Human and Animal Nutrition, 3rd ed., New York, Academic Press, pp. 323-368

US Bureau of Mines (1974) Selenium and tellurium in 1974. Mineral Industry Surveys, December 27, Washington DC, US Department of the Interior

Watkinson, J.H. (1966) Fluorometric determination of selenium in biological material with 2,3-diaminonaphthalene. Analyt. Chem., 38, 92-97

Weaver, J.N. (1973) Determination of mercury and selenium in coal by neutron activation analysis. Analyt. Chem., 45, 1950-1952

Wheeler, G.L. & Lott, P.F. (1974) Rapid determination of trace amounts of selenium (IV), nitrite and nitrate by high-pressure liquid chromatography using 2,3-diaminonaphthalene. Microchem. J., 19, 390-405

CUMULATIVE INDEX TO IARC MONOGRAPHS ON THE EVALUATION
OF CARCINOGENIC RISK OF CHEMICALS TO MAN

Numbers underlined indicate volume, and numbers in italics indicate
page. References to corrigenda are given in parentheses.

Acetamide	$\underline{7}$,*197*
Aflatoxins	$\underline{1}$,*145* (corr. $\underline{8}$,*349*)
Aflatoxin B1	$\underline{1}$,*145*
Aflatoxin B2	$\underline{1}$,*145*
Aflatoxin G1	$\underline{1}$,*145* (corr. $\underline{7}$,*319*)
Aflatoxin G2	$\underline{1}$,*145*
Aldrin	$\underline{5}$,*25*
Amaranth	$\underline{8}$,*41*
para-Aminoazobenzene	$\underline{8}$,*53*
ortho-Aminoazotoluene	$\underline{8}$,*61*
4-Aminobiphenyl	$\underline{1}$,*74*
2-Amino-5-(5-nitro-2-furyl)-1,3,4-thiadiazole	$\underline{7}$,*143*
Amitrole	$\underline{7}$,*31*
Amosite	$\underline{2}$,*17*
Aniline	$\underline{4}$,*27* (corr. $\underline{7}$,*320*)
Anthophyllite	$\underline{2}$,*17*
Apholate	$\underline{9}$,*31*
Aramite[R]	$\underline{5}$,*39*
Arsenic (inorganic)	$\underline{2}$,*48*
Arsenic pentoxide	$\underline{2}$,*48*
Arsenic trioxide	$\underline{2}$,*48*
Asbestos (mixed)	$\underline{2}$,*17* (corr. $\underline{7}$,*319*)
Auramine	$\underline{1}$,*69* (corr. $\underline{7}$,*319*)
Aziridine	$\underline{9}$,*37*
2-(1-Aziridinyl)ethanol	$\underline{9}$,*47*
Aziridyl benzoquinone	$\underline{9}$,*51*
Azobenzene	$\underline{8}$,*75*
Barium chromate	$\underline{2}$,*102*
Benz(*c*)acridine	$\underline{3}$,*241*

Benz(*a*)anthracene	<u>3</u>,*45*
Benzene	<u>7</u>,*203*
Benzidine	<u>1</u>,*80*
Benzo(*b*)fluoranthene	<u>3</u>,*69*
Benzo(*j*)fluoranthene	<u>3</u>,*82*
Benzo(*a*)pyrene	<u>3</u>,*91*
Benzo(*e*)pyrene	<u>3</u>,*137*
Beryl ore	<u>1</u>,*18*
Beryllium	<u>1</u>,*17*
Beryllium oxide	<u>1</u>,*17*
Beryllium phosphate	<u>1</u>,*25*
Beryllium sulphate	<u>1</u>,*18*
BHC (technical grades)	<u>5</u>,*47*
Bis(1-aziridinyl)morpholinophosphine sulphide	<u>9</u>,*55*
Bis(2-chloroethyl)ether	<u>9</u>,*117*
N,N'-Bis(2-chloroethyl)-2-naphthylamine	<u>4</u>,*119*
Bis(chloromethyl)ether	<u>4</u>,*231*
1,4-Butanediol dimethanesulphonate	<u>4</u>,*247*
Cadmium acetate	<u>2</u>,*92*
Cadmium powder	<u>2</u>,*74*
Cadmium carbonate	<u>2</u>,*74*
Cadmium chloride	<u>2</u>,*74*
Cadmium oxide	<u>2</u>,*74*
Cadmium sulphate	<u>2</u>,*74*
Cadmium sulphide	<u>2</u>,*74*
Calcium arsenate	<u>2</u>,*48*
Calcium arsenite	<u>2</u>,*48*
Calcium chromate	<u>2</u>,*100*
Carbon tetrachloride	<u>1</u>,*53*
Carmoisine	<u>8</u>,*83*
Chlorambucil	<u>9</u>,*125*
Chlormadinone acetate	<u>6</u>,*149*
Chlorobenzilate	<u>5</u>,*75*
Chloroform	<u>1</u>,*61*
Chloromethyl methyl ether	<u>4</u>,*239*

Chromic chromate	2,*119*
Chromic oxide	2,*100*
Chromium	2,*100*
Chromium acetate	2,*102*
Chromium carbonate	2,*102*
Chromium dioxide	2,*101*
Chromium phosphate	2,*102*
Chromium trioxide	2,*101*
Chrysene	3,*159*
Chrysoidine	8,*91*
Chrysotile	2,*17*
C.I. Disperse Yellow 3	8,*97*
Citrus Red No. 2	8,*101*
Crocidolite	2,*17*
Cycasin	1,*157* (corr. 7,*319*)
Cyclophosphamide	9,*135*
D & C Red No. 9	8,*107*
DDD (TDE)	5,*83* (corr. 7,*320*)
DDE	5,*83*
DDT	5,*83*
Diacetylaminoazotoluene	8,*113*
2,6-Diamino-3-(phenylazo)pyridine (hydrochloride)	8,*117*
Diazomethane	7,*223*
Dibenz(*a,h*)acridine	3,*247*
Dibenz(*a,j*)acridine	3,*254*
Dibenz(*a,h*)anthracene	3,*178*
7H-Dibenzo(*c,g*)carbazole	3,*260*
Dibenzo(*h,rst*)pentaphene	3,*197*
Dibenzo(*a,e*)pyrene	3,*201*
Dibenzo(*a,h*)pyrene	3,*207*
Dibenzo(*a,i*)pyrene	3,*215*
Dibenzo(*a,l*)pyrene	3,*224*
ortho-Dichlorobenzene	7,*231*
para-Dichlorobenzene	7,*231*
3,3'-Dichlorobenzidine	4,*49*

Dieldrin	_5_,125
1,2-Diethylhydrazine	_4_,153
Diethylstilboestrol	_6_,55
Diethyl sulphate	_4_,277
Dihydrosafrole	_1_,170
Dimethisterone	_6_,167
3,3'-Dimethoxybenzidine (_o_-Dianisidine)	_4_,41
para-Dimethylaminoazobenzene	_8_,125
para-Dimethylaminobenzenediazo sodium sulphonate	_8_,147
trans-2[(Dimethylamino)methylimino]-5-[2-(5-nitro-2-furyl)vinyl]-1,3,4-oxadiazole	_7_,147
3,3'-Dimethylbenzidine (_o_-Tolidine)	_1_,87
1,1-Dimethylhydrazine	_4_,137
1,2-Dimethylhydrazine	_4_,145 (corr. _7_,320)
Dimethyl sulphate	_4_,271
Endrin	_5_,157
Ethinyloestradiol	_6_,77
Ethylenethiourea	_7_,45
Ethyl methanesulphonate	_7_,245
Ethynodiol diacetate	_6_,173
Evans blue	_8_,151
2-(2-Formylhydrazino)-4-(5-nitro-2-furyl)thiazole	_7_,151
Haematite	_1_,29
Heptachlor and its epoxide	_5_,173
Hydrazine	_4_,127
4-Hydroxyazobenzene	_8_,157
Indeno(1,2,3-_cd_)pyrene	_3_,229
Iron-dextran complex	_2_,161
Iron-dextrin complex	_2_,161 (corr. _7_,319)
Iron oxide	_1_,29
Iron-sorbitol-citric acid complex	_2_,161
Isonicotinic acid hydrazide	_4_,159
Isosafrole	_1_,169
Lead acetate	_1_,40

264

Lead arsenate	<u>1</u>,*41*
Lead carbonate	<u>1</u>,*41*
Lead chromate	<u>2</u>,*101*
Lead phosphate	<u>1</u>,*48*
Lead salts	<u>1</u>,*40* (corr. <u>7</u>,*319,* <u>8</u>,*349)*
Lead subacetate	<u>1</u>,*40*
Lindane	<u>5</u>,*47*
Magenta	<u>4</u>,*57* (corr. <u>7</u>,*320)*
Maleic hydrazide	<u>4</u>,*173*
Mannomustine (dihydrochloride)	<u>9</u>,*157*
Medphalan	<u>9</u>,*167*
Medroxyprogesterone acetate	<u>6</u>,*157*
Melphalan	<u>9</u>,*167*
Merphalan	<u>9</u>,*167*
Mestranol	<u>6</u>,*87*
Methoxychlor	<u>5</u>,*193*
2-Methylaziridine	<u>9</u>,*61*
Methylazoxymethanol acetate	<u>1</u>,*164*
N-Methyl-*N*,4-dinitrosoaniline	<u>1</u>,*141*
4,4'-Methylene bis(2-chloroaniline)	<u>4</u>,*65*
4,4'-Methylene bis(2-methylaniline)	<u>4</u>,*73*
4,4'-Methylenedianiline	<u>4</u>,*79* (corr. <u>7</u>,*320)*
Methyl methanesulphonate	<u>7</u>,*253*
N-Methyl-*N*'-nitro-*N*-nitrosoguanidine	<u>4</u>,*183*
Methyl red	<u>8</u>,*161*
Methylthiouracil	<u>7</u>,*53*
Mirex	<u>5</u>,*203*
5-(Morpholinomethyl)-3-[(5-nitrofurfurylidene)amino]- 2-oxazolidinone	<u>7</u>,*161*
Mustard gas	<u>9</u>,*181*
1-Naphthylamine	<u>4</u>,*87* (corr. <u>8</u>,*349)*
2-Naphthylamine	<u>4</u>,*97*
Nickel	<u>2</u>,*126*
Nickel acetate	<u>2</u>,*126*
Nickel carbonate	<u>2</u>,*126*

Nickel carbonyl   *2*,*126* (corr. *7*,*319*)

Nickelocene   *2*,*126*

Nickel oxide   *2*,*126*

Nickel powder   *2*,*145*

Nickel subsulphide   *2*,*126*

Nickel sulphate   *2*,*127*

4-Nitrobiphenyl   *4*,*113*

5-Nitro-2-furaldehyde semicarbazone   *7*,*171*

1[(5-Nitrofurfurylidene)amino]-2-imidazolidinone   *7*,*181*

N-[4-(5-Nitro-2-furyl)-2-thiazolyl]acetamide   *1*,*181* & *7*,*185*

Nitrogen mustard (hydrochloride)   *9*,*193*

Nitrogen mustard *N*-oxide (hydrochloride)   *9*,*209*

N-Nitroso-di-*n*-butylamine   *4*,*197*

N-Nitrosodiethylamine   *1*,*107*

N-Nitrosodimethylamine   *1*,*95*

Nitrosoethylurea   *1*,*135*

Nitrosomethylurea   *1*,*125*

N-Nitroso-*N*-methylurethane   *4*,*211*

Norethisterone   *6*,*179*

Norethisterone acetate   *6*,*179*

Norethynodrel   *6*,*191*

Norgestrel   *6*,*201*

Oestradiol-17β   *6*,*99*

Oestradiol mustard   *9*,*217*

Oestriol   *6*,*117*

Oestrone   *6*,*123*

Oil orange SS   *8*,*165*

Orange I   *8*,*173*

Orange G   *8*,*181*

Phenoxybenzamine (hydrochloride)   *9*,*223*

Polychlorinated biphenyls   *7*,*261*

Ponceau MX   *8*,*189*

Ponceau 3R   *8*,*199*

Ponceau SX   *8*,*207*

Potassium arsenate   *2*,*48*

Potassium arsenite	2,*49*
Potassium chromate	2,*102*
Potassium dichromate	2,*101*
Progesterone	6,*135*
1,3-Propane sultone	4,*253*
β-Propiolactone	4,*259*
Propylthiouracil	7,*67*
Quintozene (Pentachloronitrobenzene)	5,*211*
Saccharated iron oxide	2,*161*
Safrole	1,*169*
Scarlet red	8,*217*
Selenium and selenium compounds	9,*245*
Sodium arsenate	2,*49*
Sodium arsenite	2,*49*
Sodium chromate	2,*102*
Sodium dichromate	2,*102*
Soot, tars and shale oils	3,*22*
Sterigmatocystin	1,*175*
Streptozotocin	4,*221*
Strontium chromate	2,*102*
Sudan I	8,*225*
Sudan II	8,*233*
Sudan III	8,*241*
Sudan brown RR	8,*249*
Sudan red 7B	8,*253*
Sunset yellow FCF	8,*257*
Terpene polychlorinates (Strobane[R])	5,*219*
Testosterone	6,*209*
Tetraethyllead	2,*150*
Tetramethyllead	2,*150*
Thioacetamide	7,*77*
Thiouracil	7,*85*
Thiourea	7,*95*
Trichlorotriethylamine hydrochloride	9,*229*
Tris(aziridinyl)-*para*-benzoquinone	9,*67*

267

Tris(1-aziridinyl)phosphine oxide	9,	*75*
Tris(1-aziridinyl)phosphine sulphide	9,	*85*
2,4,6-Tris(1-aziridinyl)-*s*-triazine	9,	*95*
Tris(2-methyl-1-aziridinyl)phosphine oxide	9,	*107*
Trypan blue	8,	*267*
Uracil mustard	9,	*235*
Urethane	7,	*111*
Vinyl chloride	7,	*291*
Yellow AB	8,	*279*
Yellow OB	8,	*287*
Zinc chromate hydroxide	2,	*102*

www.ingramcontent.com/pod-product-compliance
Lightning Source LLC
Chambersburg PA
CBHW081807200326
41597CB00023B/4177